Keto Diet for Beginners

Your Ultimate & Essential Step-by-Step Ketogenic Lifestyle Guide to Losing Weight Fast and Eating Better for Long-Term Weight Loss, Healthy Living and Feeling Good

Amy Maria Adams

© **Copyright 2019 by Amy Maria Adams - All rights reserved.**

The contents of this book may not be reproduced, duplicated or transmitted without direct written permission from the author.

Under no circumstances will any legal responsibility or blame be held against the publisher for any reparation, damages, or monetary loss due to the information herein, either directly or indirectly.

Legal Notice:

This book is copyright protected. This is only for personal use. You cannot amend, distribute, sell, use, quote or paraphrase any part or the content within this book without the consent of the author.

Disclaimer Notice:

Please note the information contained within this document is for educational and entertainment purposes only. Every attempt has been made to provide accurate, up to date and reliable complete information. No warranties of any kind are expressed or implied. Readers acknowledge that the author is not engaging in the rendering of legal, financial, medical or professional advice. The content of this book has been derived from various sources. Please consult a licensed professional before attempting any techniques outlined in this book.

By reading this document, the reader agrees that under no circumstances are is the author responsible for any losses, direct or indirect, which are incurred as a result of the use of information contained within this document, including, but not limited to, —errors, omissions, or inaccuracies.

Table of Contents

Introduction

Chapter 1: Getting Started with the Keto Diet for Beginners

Chapter 2: Ketogenic Diet: Common Questions Answered

Chapter 3: Keto Diet: Guidelines and Food Shopping List

Chapter 4: Simple and Easy Recipes to Start (7-Day Meal Plan)

Chapter 5: The Recipes

Chapter 6: Breakfast

Chapter 7: Soups and Salads

Chapter 8: Snacks and Side Dishes

Chapter 9: Fish and Poultry

Chapter 10: Pork and Beef

Chapter 11: Desserts and Treats

Chapter 12: The 30-Day Meal Plan

Chapter 13: How to Dine Out with the Keto Diet

Chapter 14: Mistakes to avoid when on a Keto

Diet

Bonus Chapter: Other Types of Keto Diet

Conclusion

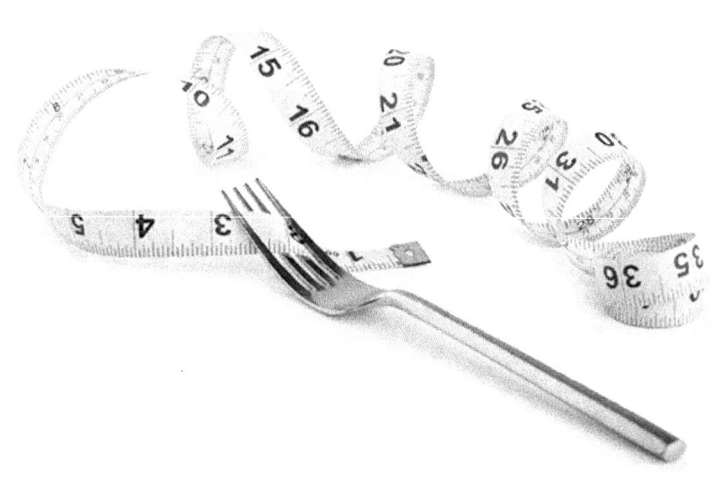

Introduction:

This book is meant to, first of all, inform you as well as serve as a guide to help you achieve that healthy lifestyle you have always desired using the ketogenic diet. The ketogenic diet is mainly natural, healthy, and at the same time, delicious. Following the ketogenic diet menu will bring about physical and mental improvements as well as help keep you energized throughout your day.

One crucial aspect of achieving success with the diet is to have a good understanding of how your body responds to food.

The keto diet was developed from fasting, which was used as a cure for epilepsy in children during the 1800s. Some believe that fasting is a cure for seizures, per the King James translation of the Bible. Mark 9:29 tells us about how Jesus cured a boy of epilepsy. When the disciples came to ask him in private why they were unable to heal (cure) the boy, Jesus stated, "this kind can come out by nothing but prayer and fasting." Notice, however, that Jesus healed the boy instantly, without recommending a fast. The most famous painting of a person with epilepsy, Raphael's *Transfiguration*, is based on this passage of scripture. The picture has two parts: the upper portion shows the transfiguration of Christ while the lower part shows the healing of the boy with epilepsy.

All kinds of diets exist—low calorie, low fat, gluten free, Weight Watchers, Atkins, South Beach, and many others. Usually, such diets entail having to starve yourself, eating uninspiring food, or being very strict about caloric intake. Many times, the challenge with these diets is that they are not nutritionally balanced and are unsatisfying. This makes them unsafe and unsustainable, meaning that you can't have a healthy lifestyle using them.

One common feature of successful diets is that they reduce foods rich in carbohydrates. Research has shown that people who eat low-fat diets and do not cut calories lose more weight than others who eat low-fat diets and also reduce calories. Also, people who eat diets low in carbohydrates usually show more improvements for important indicators like insulin and blood sugar levels, amongst many other things.

All of this depends on how your body reacts. When you eat carbohydrates, the body processes them into glucose, which is simple sugar. This leads to an increase in the levels of your blood sugar. The body then produces insulin as a way of controlling the rise in blood sugar. If you repeat this cycle over a long period, the body will naturally need to produce much more insulin at a single instance to achieve the same results.

This book will provide all you need to know to have success with the ketogenic diet. Beyond weight loss, you will learn a healthy lifestyle.

Chapter 1: Getting Started with the Keto Diet for Beginners

Chapter 1: Getting Started with the Keto Diet for Beginners

1.1 Definition of the Keto Diet

The ketogenic diet, also called the keto diet for short, is simply a diet that is high in fat and low in carbohydrates. It is also sometimes called low-carb, high-fat diet, or simply low-fat diet. The diet aims at reducing the intake of carbohydrates and replacing them with fat; this has many health advantages. By reducing the consumption of carbohydrates, the body is put in a metabolic state known as ketosis which is an increase in the number of ketone bodies in the blood.

When on a ketogenic diet, the body initiates a natural phenomenon in order to help us survive whenever food intake is low; this leads to efficiency in the way the body burns fat for energy. Also, fat is turned into ketones in the liver, which supplies energy for the brain; this is because the body is naturally adaptive to whatever is put into it. When there's an overload of fats and a reduction of carbohydrate intake, the body then begins to rely on ketones as its primary source of energy.

When not on a keto diet, the body relies on glucose as its source of energy, and therefore, fats are stored since they are not needed. The body chooses glucose over any other energy source because it is easy to convert. However, while on a keto diet, the body is deprived of that needed glucose, thereby forcing the body to depend on other sources of energy, in this case, fats. The ketogenic diet has recently become popular for weight loss amongst celebrities.

Who invented the keto diet?

Over the years, various dietary cures have been suggested for curing epilepsy, and many such treatments had to do with the increase or reduction of many substances like animals, vegetables, or minerals. Also, even though medical practitioners have adopted fasting as a mode of treatment for many sicknesses and ailments for more than two and a half thousand years now, fasting as a cure for seizures is not officially recognized.

The Hippocratic collection of the 5th Century BC

recorded fasting as its sole treatment for epilepsy. During the fifth century BC, Hippocrates wrote about a man who had an epileptic attack. Total abstinence from food and drink was the cure for the attack.

By the early twentieth century, the ketogenic diet had been used medically as a way of replicating the biochemical impacts that a fast (or starvation) would have. The earliest scientific reports that exist about the importance of fasting in epilepsy were written by French physicians Guillaume Guelpa and Auguste Marie.

It was Dr. Russell M. Wilder, an American doctor at the Mayo Clinic, that coined the term ketogenic diet.

Dr. Wilder suggested, most likely based on the work written by Woodyatt who was also a renown medical expert, "that the advantages of fasting could be acquired if ketonemia was supplied to the body by a different means. The ketone bodies are made from fat and protein at whatever point an imbalance exists between the measures of fatty acid and sugar that are consumed in the tissues. Regardless, as has for quite some time been known, it is possible to incite ketogenesis by encouraging diets which are exceptionally rich in fat and low in carbohydrates. It is proposed in this manner, to attempt the impacts of such ketogenic diets on a set of people with epilepsy." Wilder suggested that a ketogenic diet is as effective as fasting and can be sustained for a more extended period, thereby compensating for the obvious detriments of a prolonged fast.

In a report issued the next day, he depicted the surprising improvement in the seizure control of three of his epileptic patients who were admitted to the Mayo Center to be put on the ketogenic diet. He stated that, "It is difficult to reach conclusions from the results of these set of patients who were treated with high-fat diets, yet we have here a strategy for watching the impact of ketosis on the person with epilepsy. If this is the instrument responsible for the significant impact of fasting, it might be possible to substitute for that somewhat harsh method of dietary treatment which the patient can pursue with a lesser level of inconvenience and continue at their homes as long as it seems necessary."

How the ketogenic diet works

The primary source of ketone bodies for the body is via ketogenesis. The raw materials used for this process are fatty acids in adipose tissues and amino acids that are ketogenic. Adipose tissues usually serve as a site for fat storage, and this helps in the regulation of body temperature and as an energy reserve. These stored up fatty acids can be released by a hormone known as an adipokine, which is any of the several cytokines secreted by the adipose tissue, signaling that the body has a high level of glucagon and epinephrine, and hence a low insulin level. This state connotes periods of starvation or when the glucose level in the blood is low. For the metabolism of fatty acid to lead to energy production, it must occur within the mitochondria. However, free fatty acids cannot successfully transport through the biological membrane without help; this is due to the negative electric charge they carry.

As crazy as it sounds, the way the ketogenic diet works is that to lose fat, you have eat fat; this is possible because the body is put in a state of full reliance on fats where instead of storing fats, it burns fats for energy. The body is naturally programmed to run on glucose, but while on the keto diet, carbohydrate intake is very low and therefore means little glucose will be available for the body to use. Hence, the body then changes its source of energy from glucose to ketones from fats. The body becomes a fat burning machine.

What does the ketogenic diet consist of?

A ketogenic diet is a diet that contains very low carbs and very high-fat content. It shares a lot of similarities with low-carb diets and the Atkins diet. In a keto diet, fat intake is primarily replaced with carbohydrate consumption. The aim is to obtain more calories of your daily meal from protein and fat rather than from carbs.

The drastic reduction in the intake of carbohydrates makes your body begin to adapt to such changes, therefore putting your body in a metabolic state known as ketosis. When this occurs, your body becomes an efficient "fat-burning machine." Due to a massive reduction in sugar intake, the body responds to this by converting fat into ketones, to serve as an alternative source of energy for the brain, since the brain cannot utilize fat.

Who benefits from ketogenic diets?

Being on a keto diet has numerous benefits ranging from weight loss, to reduced hunger, to improved memory retention. A ketogenic diet can help in improving health conditions such as diabetes and cardiovascular disease. Usually, any diet that aids in the excessive burning of body fat and weight reduction can reduce the risk of diabetes and certain cardiovascular diseases. And, in general, any diet that helps reduce and stabilize blood glucose, keeps blood pressure in check, and reduces triglyceride levels can prevent heart disease.

What is ketosis?

Ketosis is a state in the body in which ketone bodies in the blood are used as a primary energy source, as opposed to the state in which the glucose contained in the blood serves as the primary energy source. Usually, ketosis is said to occur when the body utilizes fat at a rapid rate, leading to the conversion of fatty acids to ketones. The state of ketosis means that the body has switched from depending on carbohydrates to burning fat for fuel. As a person lessens his or her carbohydrate intake and increases dietary fats, more fat is metabolized, and ketone bodies are created. Most fats are essential to the body and do not affect heart disease risk. Fatty acids (fat) and amino acids (protein) are necessary for living. The keto diet is a low carbohydrate, high-fat diet. A standard diet is about 50 percent carbohydrates, 35 percent fat, and 15 percent protein, but the keto diet is about 70-75 percent fat, 15-20 percent protein, and about 10 percent carbohydrates. A ketogenic diet reduces the risk factor for heart diseases like stroke, epilepsy, etc. In ketosis, your body is using ketone energy for strength instead of glucose. Entering ketosis can take a little more than three days once a person begins the keto diet. At that point, a person is using fat for energy instead of carbohydrates. The keto diet promotes fresh food like meat, fish, vegetables, and healthy fat and oils. The calorie is an essential factor in the formation of ketones. A calorie is a unit of energy. Calorie consumption dictates weight gain or loss. The macronutrient is another factor in the creation of ketones. Macronutrients are found in all foods and are measured in grams (g) on nutrition labels. Fat contains nine calories per gram while protein contains four calories per gram and carbohydrates provide four calories per gram. On a keto diet, 70-75 percent of the calories one eats should come from fat.

Ketosis is a nutritional state in which the concentration of insulin (the hormone associated with fat storage) and blood glucose is at a shallow and stable level. It is associated highly with hyperketonemia, that is, an increased level of ketone bodies within the blood. Ketones, though they can be acquired through the consumption of ketone supplements, can also be produced within the body by a process known as ketogenesis in which the glycogen stored within the body is biochemically broken down. Long-term ketosis can be a result of abstaining from food or eating a low-carb diet (keto diet). Self-induced ketosis comes with medically related benefits, e.g., curing different types of diabetes, epileptic seizure reduction, appetite control, brain injury protection, athletic performance, etc.

When glucose (glycolysis) is used as the primary source of energy, insulin levels are usually at a high level, promoting fat storage, while, in ketosis, stored-up fat is typically utilized. Because of this, ketosis is sometimes called the "fat- consuming" state.

The primary ketone bodies used as an energy source are acetoacetate and beta-hydroxybutyrate. The two hormones majorly responsible for the concentration of ketone bodies in the body are glucagon and insulin. In a normal state, most cells make use of both glucose and ketone bodies for energy.

It is important to know that ketosis is entirely different from ketoacidosis, the significant difference being in the ketone levels present in the blood. Whereas ketosis is the adapting of the body to a low-carb environment, ketoacidosis, on the other hand, is life-threatening due to the alarming concentration of glucose and ketone bodies in the blood.

Abstaining from carbohydrates to the extent of ketosis is said to have both pros and cons on a person's health. Ketosis can be stimulated by periods of starvation, or after the consumption of ketone foods and supplement.

Diagnosis of ketosis

Ketosis can be detected using a specific urine test strip, for example, Ketostix and chemstrip kits.

• Ketostix are reliable for urine testing. The chemstrip is good for at least six months.

• Chemstrip kits are the second method that can be used to check urine ketones.

How to use the Ketostix

• Collect a fresh urine sample in a dry and clean container (mix the urine specimen properly before testing.)

• Perform the test in a well-lit area (any high moisture from the air will cause the strip not to work correctly.)

• Check the expiration date on the bottle of Ketostix. A new container of Ketostix can be used for six months after the first use. Always write down the day you first open the bottle on the bottle label as using the strips beyond the expiration date may lead to poor results.

• Remove one strip from the bottle. Wipe the edges of the strip along the rim of the urine container to remove excess urine. Then turn the test strip on its side and tap it once on a piece of absorbent paper.

•Hold the strip in a vertical position and compare reagent areas to the corresponding color list on the bottle label at the specified time.

• Read your results in good light.

If your test results are inconsistent or questionable:

• Check to confirm that the bottle has not expired yet as seen on the label.

• Reconfirm your result by using another Ketostix, preferably from the same container.

• Alternatively, you can also obtain a new bottle of strips and retest the specimen.

The closer the color is to deep purple, the more

ketones are in your body. Note that the test will be difficult to interpret for anyone color-blind.

Severity of ketosis

The level of ketone bodies differs based on diet, genetic influence, exercise, metabolic adaptation, etc. Ketosis can be stimulated by staying on a ketogenic diet for more than three days; this is usually referred to as "nutritional ketosis."

It is important to note that urine measurements do not equal blood measurements, as urine concentrations are usually more hydrated and therefore lower. After staying on a ketogenic diet for a while, the concentration lost in the urine may be reduced while the metabolism still relies on ketone bodies in the blood as an energy supply. Blood tests for ketones are much more reliable; however, the test strips are costly. Urine ketone testing is notoriously unreliable.

Most urine strips only detect acetoacetate levels, while, in a severe case of ketosis, the predominant ketone body will be beta-hydroxybutyrate. At any blood level, ketones are excreted into the urine; this is quite the opposite when it comes to glucose. Ketoacidosis is a disorder that can't take place within a healthy individual who secretes insulin normally.

Controversies about ketosis

Some health experts consider abstinence from carbohydrate diets unhealthy. However, achieving a state of ketosis does not require the complete elimination of carbohydrates from the menu. Other health experts regard ketosis as a simple metabolic process that is characterized by fat-burning. Ketosis, which is usually followed by gluconeogenesis, is the particular state that worries some health experts. However, it is rare for a person in good health to reach a dangerous keto level. Individuals who suffer from the inability to secrete basal insulin are more likely to reach a life-threatening level of ketosis, eventually leading to a coma.

Signs and symptoms that can help you know if you are in ketosis

You can monitor your ketosis level using a urine or blood strip, but these are quite expensive. Alternatively, you can use specific "markers" to know if you've got it right:

- **Frequent urination** – The keto diet is a diuretic and therefore increases the rate of urine excretion. Acetoacetate, a ketone body, is usually excreted with urine.
- **Dry mouth** – the increased urination usually leads to an increase in thirst and a dry mouth. Hence, ensure you stay hydrated in order to regulate your electrolytes.
- **Mouth odor** – acetone is a ketone body that smells like an overripe fruit; it is released when we breathe. This odor gradually is reduced over the long-term.
- **Curbs hunger levels and increase energy** – a reduced hunger level usually characterizes the ketosis state.

Discomforts you may suffer during the first few weeks of being in ketosis

Your body is already well familiar with the normal process of utilizing carbohydrates as an energy source. Over time, the body secretes myriad enzymes to assist this process, but only a few enzymes associated with the breaking down of fat.

And all of a sudden, your body has to adapt to

the reduction in glucose level and increase in total fat intake, which means having to build up an entirely different arsenal of enzymes. As your body initiates a state of ketosis, your body will utilize its remaining glucose reserve, breaking down glycogen in the muscles, which can cause a reduction in performance and lack of energy.

During the first week, many individuals complain of dizziness, headaches, etc. This is usually the side effects of the loss of most of your electrolytes, as ketosis increases the rate of urine excretion. These can be countered by drinking plenty of water and increasing your salt intake.

Sodium will aid with water retention and assist in replenishing flushed-out electrolytes.

What is a macro? And how to measure it?

Macros, also known as macronutrients, are fats, proteins, and carbohydrates. They play a vital role in providing our body with essential nutrients and acting as a primary energy source for our daily activities; this is what earns them the term "macro," meaning "large." We not only need them for the proper functioning of our body system, but we also need them to live.

Macro-measuring means to measure the macronutrients in your diet to ensure you're consuming the ideal daily amount of fats, proteins, and carbohydrates, although the perfect amount of each differs from individual to individual depending on certain factors like lifestyle, metabolism, and age. In other words, when measuring your macros, you will need to understand your body and what it needs. Knowing your body well may take a bit of time, but it's worth it.

How to measure macro?

They are measured in percentages, so it's not necessary to count calories; you only need to estimate what percent of each of these macros you have in your food; this makes consuming whole foods much easier since their macro content is easy to obtain. This is not the same with processed foods, whose macro-measurement is a little trickier, but not impossible. You will have to do a more in-depth label reading to find out what the food that you want to eat contains.

When macro-measuring, it is not necessary to count; you only need to measure macros. Look at everything you consume like it's a pie, and the content of each macro is a slice.

For example, your meal may contain the following; 40 percent carbs, 30 percent fats, and 30 percent protein. This is very standard and is very suitable for middle-aged individuals with an average rate of metabolism. This means that 40 percent of your daily "pie" allocation must come from carbohydrates, 30 percent from fat, and 30 percent from protein. This means that as you eat daily, you should calculate the macro percentages. This doesn't have to be an exact science; just take mental stock of what you eat and then deduct it from your daily percentage allowance.

Thanks to the advent of the internet, you can easily use the Keto Online Calculator to calculate macros. You can access such calculator at www.ketovale.com/keto-calculator/, www.keto-calculator.ankerl.com/, www.ketokarma.com/keto-calculator and many websites available online. These websites take your body type and activity level into consideration, so you can rest assured that they're quite correct.

Understand your body

Your sex and age play a minor role in determining your exact macro requirements. Your body type is the primary factor that affects and determines your macro requirements. You have to understand your metabolism, which is your physiological self, to achieve accurate macro measurements. In general, we have three body types. They include:

• **Ectomorph** – this body type is slender, with a small bone structure, and gaining weight and muscle mass can be difficult. An individual in this category will require a macro constituent of 50-60 percent carbs, 30-40 percent protein, and 20-30 percent fat.

• **Mesomorph** – this body type is naturally strong and muscular, with broad shoulders and very dense bones. Gaining or losing weight is moderately easy, while gaining muscle mass is very easy. Individuals in this category will require a macro constituent of 40-50 percent carbs, 35-45 percent protein, and 25-35 percent fat.

• **Endomorphs** – this body type is stocky, involving a round body and shorter limbs. Gaining muscle mass is very easy, but losing weight is extremely hard. Individuals in this category will require a macro constituent of 20-30 percent carbs, 30-40 percent fat, and 50-60 percent protein.

Even after understanding how your body functions, you will still have to adjust your macros to suit your goals and daily activity level. In general, if your goal is to burn fat and gain muscle, your protein percentage should be the highest. Your carb intake should be the lowest, and your fat intake should remain moderate.

1.2 Benefits of keto diets

The ketogenic diet differs from other diets in the sense that many of those diets offer weight loss as their main advantage. The ketogenic diet comes with a large number of benefits because of the way it alters the chemical composition of the body. The keto diet leads to an increase in the production of ketones, as well as a dependence on ketones for the daily maintenance of the body. The body is more efficient when it depends on ketones as fuel. Amongst the many advantages of the ketogenic diet, a few will be discussed below:

- **Weight loss** – because of its low carbohydrate content, the ketogenic diet brings about a breaking down of body fat into ketones and allows the body to depend mainly on ketones rather than glucose. In other words, the fat stored up in the body will be used as a source of energy. When an individual is on a keto diet, insulin, which is the fat-storing hormone level, drops massively, turning the body into a fat-consuming machine since fat storage is prevented. Scientifically, on long-term analysis, a regularly practiced ketogenic diet has proven to show better results as compared to low-fat and high-carb diets; cholesterol is produced from the conversion of excess glucose in the diet. Ketogenic diets generally have an improved feeling of satiety, hence leading to an overall reduction in food intake. This allows for reduced calorie intake without necessarily causing ravenous hunger.

• **Reversion of nephropathy** – nephropathy is one of the complications associated with individuals who have uncontrolled diabetes. Studies have shown that keto diets aid the reversing of diabetic nephropathy by increasing the level of 3-beta-hydroxybutyric acid in the blood, which leads to the subsequent reduction in the metabolism of glucose in some tissues within the body, for example, the kidneys. In a study performed by Poplawski et al., during one week of administering the ketogenic diets to rats, the glucose level in the blood normalized. Within two months, the albumin/creatinine ratio was also standardized, and diabetic nephropathy was completely reversed. This is associated with the expression of genes induced by oxidation and various forms of stress being normalized. In a human, the ketogenic diet causes a decrease in the level of creatinine as compared to the consumption of low-calorie foods, which show an increase in the level of creatinine. Ketones can serve as an alternative source of energy.

- **Boost brain health** – the brain, unlike the muscles, cannot utilize fat as a source of energy; therefore, the brain is heavily dependent on glucose. The brain, however, can utilize ketones. The liver uses fatty acid to produce ketones in situations where glucose and insulin levels are low. Ketones are usually produced in little amounts when one hasn't eaten for long hours, for example, after a full night's sleep. However, the liver's production of ketones increases during periods of fasting, starvation, or when the level of carb intake is below 50 g per day. When the consumption of carbs is minimized, ketones can cater for up to 70 percent of the brain's needs. Although most of the brain can utilize ketones, some parts depend solely on glucose for their functionality. When one is on a low-carb diet, some of this glucose can be provided for by the small intake of carbs. The body, however, synthesizes most of the glucose requirements in a process known as gluconeogenesis. In this metabolic process, the liver produces glucose for the brain to utilize; it uses amino acids as its raw material. The liver can also produce glucose from glycerol; this is the backbone that connects fatty acids in triglyceride molecules—the body's form of storing fat. Staying on a ketogenic diet has been proven to be effective against Parkinson's disease as well. It is most likely that certain features associated with remaining on a ketogenic diet, such as an increase in brain sharpness, mental clarity, and less frequent migraines are related to the controlled level of sugar in the blood serum and change of energy source for the brain, which helps improve memory.

- **Increase in the levels of HDL cholesterol** – whenever people hear about an increase in the level of cholesterol, there is usually a panic, and this is because many are not well informed that there are two types of cholesterol (the HDL and the LDL). The HDL is the one that is more needed because it carries cholesterol from the body to the liver (the liver is where it can be reused or excreted.) Conversely, the LDL transports cholesterol from the liver to all parts of the body.

- **Reduction of epileptic seizures** – seizures are a complication associated with epilepsy. It usually manifests as continuous jerking movements and fainting; it occurs mostly in children. Epilepsy is tough to treat. There are several types of seizures. Although many effective anti-seizure medications exist, these drugs are usually ineffective in at least 30 percent of epilepsy patients. This type of epilepsy is known as "unresponsive to medication." The ketogenic diet, developed by Dr. Russell Wilder in 1921, supplies the body with about 90 percent of calories from fat and is effective in treating drug-resistant epilepsy in children, as it has been said to imitate the important effects that starvation has on seizures. The particular mechanism, however, remains unknown, but it is believed to help in increasing the stability of neurons and regulation of mitochondrial enzymes.
- **Beneficial for individuals with Alzheimer's disease** – ketogenic diets provide benefits to people with Alzheimer's disease. Alzheimer's is a gradually advancing

disease in which the brain develops tangles that result in loss of memory. Many researchers believe that it should be classified as "type 3" diabetes because the brain cells develop insulin resistance and lack the ability to utilize glucose properly, causing inflammation. Health experts claim that Alzheimer's disease has certain common features with epilepsy, for example, overexcitement of the brain cells that leads to seizures. It has been suggested that ketogenic diets may be an effective method of fueling brain cells affected by Alzheimer's disease. One hypothesis is that ketone bodies protect the cells of the brain by limiting the level of reactive oxygen species which are by-products of metabolism that may cause inflammation. Another hypothesis states that the lethal proteins that accumulate in the brains of individuals with Alzheimer's disease can be reduced by a diet that contains a high amount of fat.

• **Battling cancer** – cancerous cells express a metabolism that is different from the metabolism of healthy cells. They are usually characterized by rapid increase in glucose utilization. This is due to the many insulin receptors in them, causing them to thrive in an environment that has high levels of both insulin and blood sugar, usually caused by mutations and mitochondrial dysfunction. Cancerous cells, unlike healthy cells, cannot effectively utilize ketone bodies as an energy source. Also, ketone bodies restrain the proliferation of tumor cells, and they can provide energy for healthy cells without feeding the tumor cells. Ketogenic diets, however, can only be helpful against some types of cancer.

• **Boosts energy levels and improves sleep** – after staying on a ketogenic diet for about four to five days, most individuals experience an increase in energy levels and a general lack of interest in carbohydrate diets; this is as a result of a readily available energy source and the insulin level being stabilized in body and brain tissues. When placed on a low-carb diet, the body can only store so much glycogen, and as a result, constant refueling is necessary to maintain energy levels. However, your body already has as alternative fat storage to utilize; this means that ketosis is a source of fuel to the body that can never be exhausted and you'll find that you have energy throughout the day. The mechanism of sleep improvement remains a mystery. However, studies have shown that staying on a ketogenic diet helps improve sleep by reducing REM and increasing slow-wave sleep patterns. This is most likely related to the biochemical shifts associated with the brain now depending on ketone bodies as an alternate energy source and other body tissues breaking down fat. However, during the first few weeks of staying on a ketogenic diet (the adjustment period), you may experience particular difficulties in staying asleep and insomnia. This will wane with time as your body becomes accustomed to ketosis and to consuming stored-up fat. And then you'll find that you feel more relaxed, can sleep deeply for more hours, and feel rested when you wake.

• **Aids kidney functions** – kidney stones and gout are mostly caused by an increase in uric acid, phosphate, and calcium levels. This is as a result of obesity, dehydration, consumption of sugar (especially fructose), and alcohol consumption. Uric acid levels can be temporarily increased by ketogenic diets, especially when a person is dehydrated, though its level decreases over time. Uric acid levels increase within the same time frame as ketone bodies, but after a period of four to six weeks, uric acid levels begin to decrease despite ketone levels staying up. Hence, the individual might have a low uric acid level despite being in a state of nutritional ketosis.

• **Helping women's health** – polycystic ovary syndrome (PCOS) can be effectively treated with low-carbohydrate diets which help to stop specific symptoms such as obesity, infrequent menstrual periods, and acne. Keto diets also help in keeping the level of sugar in the blood serum deficient and stabilized. They also help to maintain the level of other hormones, and especially in women, this has a lot of benefits in a wide variety of metabolic pathways associated with insulin.

• **Helps battle type 2 diabetes** – individuals

that suffer from type 2 diabetes exhibit excessive insulin production. Because keto diets are low-carb and hence remove sugar from the food, they assist in the reduction of the HbA1c count. That can, therefore, help reverse type 2 diabetes. Ketogenic diets also help in reversing nephrology, provide cardiac benefits, assist with weight loss, and improve lipid profiles.

• **Helps boost gastrointestinal health and liver health** – it is common knowledge that grain-based foods, nightshade vegetables (such as tomatoes, potatoes, etc.), and sugar-filled foods increase the chances of heartburn and acid reflux. It is, therefore, of little surprise that maintaining a low-carb diet helps improve these symptoms, confronting the problems of autoimmune responses and inflammation. With regards to this, changes in diet alter the total human gut microbiome (you are what you eat). A variation in the microbiome substantially reduces most gastrointestinal problems as a result of staying on the ketogenic diet. Studies have shown that carbs in the diet are highly associated with gallstones as they are the main ingredients that cause them. As a countereffect, eating an appropriate amount of fat when carb intake is down assists in the clearing out of the gallbladder and improves functionality, thus reducing the chances of gallstones forming. Fat accumulating in the liver is related to prediabetes and type 2 diabetes; in very extreme cases, fatty liver disease can be very lethal to the liver. This condition is usually tested using a blood test to measure the level of liver enzymes.

• **Decreases inflammation** – ketogenic diets are highly anti-inflammatory and help in improving a lot of health problems. The anti-inflammatory properties of ketogenic diets, or a reduction in caloric intake, may be linked to retardation of the hormone responsible for inflammation. In other words, the main ingredients responsible for most inflammatory diseases are repressed by ketone bodies made from a ketogenic diet. Thus, its effect on acne, psoriasis, eczema, arthritis, and other inflammation-associated diseases is reasonably significant enough to attract more research attention. It is, therefore, very possible to improve a whole host of conditions through nutritional ketosis.

• **Helps in appetite control** – when staying on a low-carb diet, you'll find that you don't feel hungry as often as before; you don't develop random cravings that make you go on an excessive snacking spree and cause you to eat bad things. Many individuals that stay on a ketogenic diet find it easier to perform intermittent fasting, where you're feeding not as consistently as before, and you only get to eat at certain set periods of the day. Controlling the sugar level in the blood can help with curbing such cravings and uncontrollable appetites.

This book will help every newbie understand the keto diet; there are recipes within the book to try out which will improve your health and well-being.

1.3

One of the ways you can find out how much you know, do not know or need to know about the keto diet as a beginner and is to take online tests. That's a good way of checking your knowledge base (if it's sound enough) and there are many websites where you can take such tests. You can take tests at "Completely Keto" at http://completelyketo.com or "Bhu Foods" at http://bhufoods.com

Your Quick Start Action Step:

Create some time before the end of the day to take the test at any of the websites listed above and take the tests.

None of the tests should take more than 15 to 20 minutes.

Chapter 2: The Ketogenic Diet – Common Questions Answered

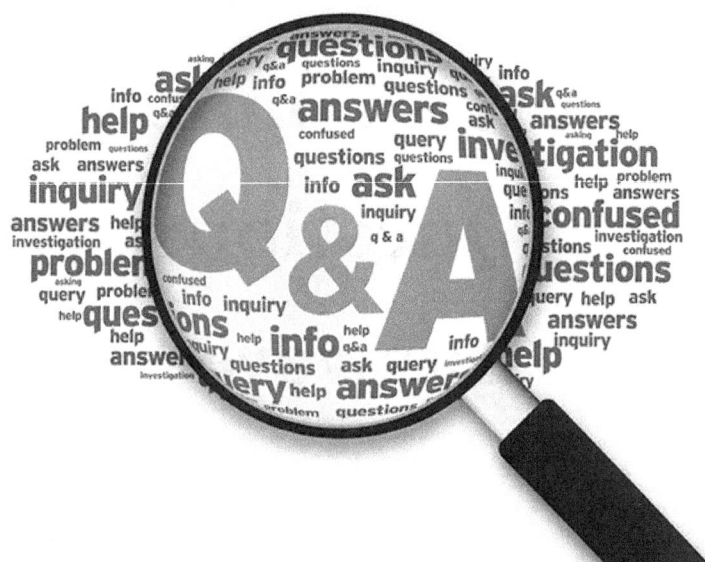

Chapter 2: The Ketogenic Diet – Common Questions Answered

2.1 Is the ketogenic diet safe?

It is normal that whenever a new diet hits the scene, there's always information that talks about its negative impacts on your health. However, what is the case with the keto diet? The keto diet has undergone scientific tests and analysis and has been recommended by great medical institutions globally. It has been proven to be safe; however, this depends on the activity level and condition of the individual. But on a general scale, it is entirely safe. It is helpful for achieving a healthy lifestyle and not just a miracle cure.

2.2 Does the ketogenic diet work?

The ketogenic diet has been in use for a very long time; it became more pronounced in the 1920s and since then has been used repeatedly on different individuals. The keto diet started as a cure for epileptic children, with many of them being completely cured. The ketogenic diet has been proven to work for many conditions starting from weight loss to heart disease. Its impact on weight loss has been debated as a short-term impact; some patients apparently regain weight after about a year or two. But this is highly debatable.

2.3 Does the ketogenic diet work for the long-term?

It is highly debatable whether the use of ketogenic diets for weight loss works for the long-term; however, it is not medically or scientifically proven otherwise. Using weight loss for other diseases works, for example, for people with diabetes, and the cure is long-term. The same thing applies to high-blood pressure if they are able to follow through with the diet successfully.

2.4 Does the ketogenic diet affect weight loss?

The answer is yes. The ketogenic diet is gaining popularity again not precisely because of its benefits for other diseases but because of its use for weight loss. The ketogenic diet is beneficial for weight loss because of the dramatic reduction in the intake of carbohydrates, forcing the body to burn fat as its source of energy rather than glucose from carbohydrates. It also reduces appetite, which also contributes to weight loss. By affecting appetite, it reduces individuals' cravings for sugar.

2.5 How does a ketogenic diet affect cholesterol?

It is a common misconception that since ketogenic diets are high in fat content, they lead to an increase in cholesterol levels in the body. However, this is not true. Much scientific research has shown that low-carb diets help in optimizing the cholesterol level in the body. Many are unaware that there is good cholesterol and bad cholesterol. HDL cholesterol is the one known as "the good cholesterol." It collects all cholesterol that is not in use within the body and takes it to the liver, where it is either recycled or destroyed. The ketogenic diet causes a reduction in LDL, "the bad cholesterol," which is responsible for some cardiovascular diseases in adults.

2.6 What is the "keto flu" and how do you minimize it?

Starting a keto diet can be very strange. You have a lot to look forward to including a lot of weight loss and a lot of anticipated internal changes that your body is bound to undergo. However, keto flu is something else that might also come along when starting a keto diet. Your body may experience keto flu during the initial stages of being on a keto diet. Usually, the body gets a little weak before it finally starts getting stronger. The extent to which your body suffers usually depends largely on your previous diet as it determines the shock your system will undergo from your new diet pattern; the effect of that shock is what you will begin to experience.

Once you start a keto diet, some symptoms are sure markers of having the keto flu. They include:

- Headaches

- A cough

- Fatigue

- Irritability

- Nausea

These symptoms are usually indications that your body needs to adjust to the changes in your diet pattern and adapt to what you're putting it through. Having these symptoms is not enjoyable, and it sucks; they can leave you discouraged and make you wonder whether it is worth the pain and discomfort. However, these symptoms will eventually fade away as your body approaches ketosis. These symptoms are just your body reacting to carb deprivation, but over time, these symptoms will go just as quickly as they came.

A ketogenic diet contains a very low-carb content, and therefore your body tries to adapt to the low intake of carbs since you have been consuming a large amount of carbs your whole life up to this point. Staying away from carbs will tend to come as a shock to your body, but very soon your body will recover and continues on the path to good health. When suffering from the keto flu, you may start to consider eating more carbs to make the pain and discomfort go away, but do not listen to this temptation; endure for a couple of days, and everything will go back to normal.

How to minimize the flu?

Once on a keto diet, one of the numerous changes your body will undergo is a loss of body fluids and electrolytes in the form of sodium, potassium, and magnesium. Electrolytes are vital to the proper functioning of your body as they play a significant role in determining the amount of water in your body and how effectively your muscles perform their task. Carbs usually help with water retention within the body, ensuring there is no excessive loss of electrolytes. When staying on a keto diet, you will begin to lose a lot of body fluids, and since most electrolytes are dissolved in these fluids as a solvent, it is natural that you will lose some of them. Also, since your body is going to be consuming a lot of stored-up body fat, and your body cells will begin to replace these fats with water, it is essential to stay hydrated. It is also necessary to add a lot of salt to your daily meal by eating foods that have a high sodium content. If your electrolyte consumption is high, then you'll be just fine.

How long will it take for my body to adjust?

When on a regular diet, your body is, necessarily, sugar dependent but when on a keto diet, your body becomes fat dependent. This kind of change usually has a drastic effect on the body, but time is all your body requires. The adjustment period differs with individuals. However, on average, it takes more than a week to finally reach the ketosis stage; for some, it occurs faster than that. It all depends on how your body reacts to the effect of such changes; this is the time your body begins to shed some fat. It is essential to note that even when your body has reached the ketosis stage, that doesn't mean it will stay in it when you begin to eat carbs again. Some individuals can get away with it; others can't. It is just safer to adhere strictly to your diet.

2.7 How many carbs can I eat on the keto diet?

The amount of carbs every individual needs is dependent on a couple of things. Generally, eating less carbs has more impact. It will speed weight loss and reduce appetite and hunger. Someone with type 2 diabetes should eat fewer carbohydrates; it will improve insulin resistance. The truth is that many people find a diet that is very low in carbs somewhat too challenging and restrictive.

2.8 How much protein should I eat on the keto diet?

When on a keto diet, it is essential to eat a lot of protein. However, if you eat too much of it, this will lower your ketone levels; if you eat too little, it leads to you losing excess muscle. So you should be at the midpoint in that sense. For someone that is sedentary, that is, you do a whole lot of sitting during the day, you should eat around 0.6 grams and 0.8 grams of protein for every pound of lean body mass. If you are someone who has an active day, you should eat between 0.8 grams and one gram of protein for every pound of lean body mass. If you want to gain some muscle, you should eat about one gram and 1.2 grams of protein for every pound of lean body mass. You don't need more protein than that.

2.9 What ketogenic diet is best?

In selecting the best diet, there are some things to consider. If you're someone who rarely engages in highly intense exercise and wants to lose weight, you should stick to the standard keto diet. If you add more carbohydrates, you will only be slowing down your progress and prolong how long it takes to reach ketosis, unlike those who don't add carbs. For people who engage in intense exercise regularly, then the cyclical keto diet and the targeted keto diet might be right for you. If you're someone who has only started intense workouts regularly within the last year, you should try out the targeted keto diet and see if you notice a decrease in performance while you're on the standard keto diet. When it comes to figuring out the best type of keto diet for you, it is important that you experiment. There are no individuals that are the same; you must find out what works for you best. It is important also to note that if you're not doing intense exercise regularly, then you should stay on the standard keto diet. Usually, most people do not need anything more than the standard keto diet.

Chapter 3: Keto Diet – Guidelines and Food Shopping List

FRUITS
Let fruits jazz up your feast!

Apples
Avocado
Bananas
Blueberries
Cranberries
Grapefruit

Olive
Sunflower

Chapter 3: Keto Diet – Guidelines and Food Shopping List

3.1 Guidelines for the ketogenic diet

Find out what you need to eat and avoid while on the diet

To follow a keto diet meal plan or food list, you'll be reducing carbs on a diet. You should start by eating about 20 to 30 grams of carbs per day. You should do some research and find out food items that are mostly carbs, protein, and fats; this will help you make the right choices. Examples of foods that are high in carbs are not just limited to pasta, bread, cookies, chips, candy, and ice cream. Most fruits and vegetables also contain mostly carbs. The only foods that have zero carbs are meat (protein) and pure fats like oil and margarine.

Examine your love for fat

Keto diets involve a whole lot of fats, so you

must love them. Many are scared of eating fats because they have been told it will kill them. Before starting the keto diet, begin by adjusting your daily food intake to accommodate high fats; you can substitute green vegetables for fries or order a burger on lettuce leaves. Rather than rice or potatoes, you can eat a non-starchy vegetable. Cook with more oil. Slowly introduce fats into your meals and reduce the carb content. The keto diet won't work for you if you're the type that is scared of fats.

Sharpen your cooking abilities

You need to sharpen your cooking skills as high-carb processed foods are a no-go area while on a diet. You must learn how to make fresh meals. You can have a look at the sample recipes in the later chapters of this book, and you'll fall in love with them. Check out recipes you know you will like online as well. By doing this, you will lessen the chances of having to revert to carbs.

Try keto-friendly drinks

You should try bulletproof coffee. It's one of the greatest warm keto beverages. It's made by just mixing butter and coconut oil with your coffee. This drink reduces hunger levels, thereby allowing you extra time to plan your next meal properly.

A note of caution: if you have heart disease, then you might want to avoid this drink. For safety's sake, you should ask your doctor if it is safe for you.

Speak with your family about your goals on the diet

Clearly state your plan. You will not be able to eat all meals with them, so you will have to make your meals yourself. Sometimes, there might be an objection. Explain that you have adequately researched the diet, have found it to be safe, and want to try this out.

Clean out your pantry

When you decide to go on the keto diet, one of the first things to do is to discard everything that is anti-keto. Keeping tempting but unhealthy foods around your home can be the biggest cause of failure for your keto diet. Hence, to achieve success, you must reduce such temptations to a bearable minimum. Unless you are very strong-willed, you shouldn't keep tempting foods such as desserts, loaves of bread very high in sugar, and other anti-keto snacks around you.

If you're the kind of person who lives with others, ensure you inform your housemates and family members, as well as other people you live with, and warn them before throwing anything out of the house. If some food items must be hidden (that is, if they're not yours and can't be thrown out), you all should agree about a good place where they can be out of sight. Doing this will make it clear to those you live with that you are pretty serious about your new diet, and will ultimately result in a great experience for you at home. It is normal for people to want to tempt you when you start a new diet, but eventually, as time passes, they'll stop.

Some of the things you should keep away include;

Sugary foods and drinks: You need to get rid

of all processed sugar, fruit juices, desserts, pastries, fountain drinks, milk, milk chocolate, candy bars, etc.

Fruits: Get rid of all fruits that have a high-carb content; this includes apples, mangoes, dates, bananas, and grapes. You must ensure you rid yourself of all dried fruits like raisins, too. Dried fruits usually have as much sugar as regular fruits, but they're even more concentrated which makes it easy to consume a whole lot of sugar in small servings. For instance, a cup of raisins contains 100 grams of carbohydrates; meanwhile, a cup of grapes contains about 15 grams of carbs.

Starches and grains: You should get rid of all types of cereal, rice, corn, rolls, pasta, wraps, oats, bread, quinoa, bagels, flour, potatoes, and croissants.

Processed polyunsaturated fats and oils: Get rid of most seed oils. Seed oils to eliminate include safflower, corn oil, grapeseed, sunflower, and canola. Also, get rid of trans fats like margarine and shortening—anything that reads "hydrogenated," even if it's partial. The kind of oils you should keep at home are coconut oil, olive oil, avocado oil, and extra-virgin olive oil. These are the keto-friendly ones.

Legumes: You should also get rid of beans, lentils, and peas. They are highly concentrated with carbs. A typical one-cup serving of beans contains three times more carbs than you should consume in a day.

Don't miss the point: you are meant to get rid of all keto-unfriendly food items, but these foods are still good for others. Hence, you shouldn't throw them into the trash can; other people can eat them. Look for people around you to whom you can donate them. Your pantry should look empty after you clean it out; this is because most of the food items that can be stored for the long-term are usually high in carbs and usually contain unhealthy preservatives and additives.

Kitchen utensils to use

Having the right low-carb kitchen gadgets can make life a little easier and your diet more successful. You shouldn't waste money on kitchen utensils that are unnecessary. Some of them might be things you have in your kitchen already.

- **Kitchen Scales**

Kitchen scales are important for measuring out menu sizes for beginners. Without kitchen scales, it will be hard to know the macronutrient size of your food since you can't say how much you eat. The keto diet requires that you cook by weight. It is entirely accurate, and there is no room for error. Recipe failures are sometimes because people cook by volume (that is, using cups). They usually fill their cups too firmly or too loosely, thereby leading to adding too much or too little of an ingredient or food item, making the recipe a disaster. Start using electronic scales and save yourself some trouble. You can easily switch between ounces or grams, depending on what you want. Making use of scales also reduces your washing up. Zero the scales, add your first food item, zero the scales again, and then add your second item, etc.

- **Slow Cooker**

This is perfect for making recipes while you're on the go. Set it before you leave and forget it!

The slow cooker is a great utensil. It makes life easier. If you know you have a crazy day ahead and won't be home until late after sports and other activities are finished, always put on the slow cooker. By the time you walk in the door, dinner will already be waiting.

- **Frying Pan/Skillet**

Try to buy one with a heavy base so the heat is well distributed and steady. You will notice the difference.

One utensil to love is the electric frying pan. If you want to cook a big breakfast for a family of five, you have to squeeze in bacon, eggs, greens, and tomatoes. That is the way to conveniently cook a full meal in one go.

The eggs cook perfectly with the lid on, the bacon doesn't dry up, and they all remain warm if you're still in the shower when breakfast is ready. No more messing up two frying pans or keeping things warm in the oven.

- **Spiralizers (Handheld, Benchtop)**

Vegetable noodles are popular and are a better/healthier substitute for pasta.

Handheld spiralizers are very easy to take along on holiday with you but can be a little slower to use, and you need to keep your little fingers away from the exposed sharp blades lest they cut you.

The benchtop spiralizer is the fast one. Plus, it's fun for the children to use. It is very safe and washes easily. It comes with different three blades to create varied sized ribbons of "pasta" or noodles.

- **Stick Blender**

I recommend buying a stick blender with multiple attachment options. You can use the mini processor to grind nuts and almonds, and the whisk to whip cream.

- **Food Processor**

This is another kitchen utensil that you must have for pureeing and chopping.

It can be used for grating/shredding carrots for making low-carb carrot cake, and it's great for cheese, because buying pre-grated/shredded cheese will cost you a whole lot more. You can also use it for making a flourless orange cake.

• **Measuring Cups And Spoons**

These are important for the same reason as the kitchen scale. If you want to know exactly what your servings are, measuring cups and spoons help you to do this. Also, measuring correctly enables you to achieve better-tasting recipes!

• **Mixing Bowls, Various Sizes**

You can choose to buy stackable mixing bowls to save space in your cupboards. If you can find those with lids, they can also be used for storage in the fridge.

• **Baking Trays, Cake Pans**

Loose-bottom cake pans can be used for chocolate heaven cake and lemon coconut cake to ensure it cooks evenly.

• **Roasting Pan**

One great meal you can always have is roasted meat and vegetables. It can be prepared on a regular basis.

You can put two roasting pans in the oven every time. One for the vegetables and meat, and another for preparing your grain-free granola.

- **Parchment Paper, Non-Stick Baking Sheets/Silicone Mat**

These are important for preparing some recipes like the Fat head pizza as well as to line cake pans.

Ensure you have these so you don't difficulties cleaning up when you're done cooking or baking.

- **Knives**

You should have a good solid knife set in your kitchen. They can make all the difference.

They'll make your cooking safer, faster, and easier.

- **Mortar And Pestle**

You will be doing some grinding. You can use a mortar and pestle to grind granulated sweetener in case you run out.

A powdered sweetener is an essential ingredient for making sugar-free chocolate shells; also, it is easier to add it to fat bombs or fudge.

- **Waffle Maker And Coffee Maker**

These are not so important, but can make your keto life nicer.

- **Egg Cooker**

If you love eating eggs, then you should have one of these. They can poach or boil many eggs at a time.

Having an egg cooker is a good choice if you have to cook some boiled eggs for school lunches for the next day. This will save you from having to go to the grocery store numerous times.

- **Food-Prep Bowls With Covers, And Storage Containers**

You will need to have storage containers. You will need as many as you can use to keep a couple of meals in the fridge, including any leftovers.

It's also good to have a range of tiny containers to put leftovers in so you can add them to school lunchboxes in the morning. Nothing should go to waste.

• **Kids' Lunchboxes**

If you want to be a real food family who has ditched the junk food and processed food, you'll need a decent lunchbox.

• **Silicon Cupcake Cases**

These are awesome for cooking and perfect for lunchboxes.

Not only are these great for making low-carb cupcakes, but they are also handy for serving berries in a lunchbox or little cheese cubes, setting mini Jell-Os, or making fat bombs. You should have silicon cupcake cases in a variety of shapes.

• **Ice-Cream Makers**

For regular ice cream, it is not essential to have

an ice-cream maker. But having an ice-cream maker makes a lovely, light, and fluffy scoop.

Shopping list

Below is a comprehensive list of what a shopping list should include; the carb content for each food item is also mentioned to help you make an informed decision. Eating less carbs can have amazing medical benefits. It has been proven to diminish general hunger levels, which will, in turn, lead to dramatic weight loss without having to keep checking your calorie intake.

About 23 studies have shown that low-carb diets can cause up to two times more weight loss than low-fat diets. Eating low-carb doesn't need to be technical.

To get thinner and improve your health, just make sure your diet contains natural foods that are low in carbs. Listed below are some low-carb foods that should be found on your keto shopping list, all of which are nutritious, healthy, and unimaginably delicious.

The amount of carbs for a standard serving, and the number of carbs in a 100-gram serving, are listed toward the end of each segment.

In any case, remember that some of these foods have very high fiber content, which may reduce the absorbable net carb.

Meats and Eggs

Eggs, and a wide range of beef, are near zero carbs. Organ meats are a peculiar case. For example, liver contains about five percent carbs.

- **Eggs (almost zero)**

Eggs are some of the most beneficial and nutritional foods on earth. They contain different nutrients—including some that are essential for your mind— and can enhance the health of your eyes. Eggs have almost zero carbs.

- **Beef (zero)**

Beef is profoundly satisfying and full of essential nutrients like iron and vitamin B12. There are many diverse kinds of beef, from ground beef to ribeye steak to hamburger. Beef contains zero carbs.

• Lamb (zero)

Like beef, lamb contains numerous advantageous nutrients, including iron and vitamin B12. Lamb is regularly grass-nourished, and will, in general, be high in the essential fatty acid conjugated linoleic acid (CLA). Lamb has zero carbs.

• Chicken (zero)

Chicken is among the world's most common meats. It's high in numerous helpful nutrients and a fantastic source of protein. In case you're on a low-carb diet, it might be a good decision to go for fattier cuts like wings and thighs. Chicken has zero carbs.

• Pork, including Bacon (usually zero)

Pork is another tasty kind of meat, and bacon is the most loved protein for numerous low-carb dieters. Bacon is processed meat, and consequently might not be so healthy. Be that as it may, it's generally acceptable to eat reasonable amounts of bacon on a low-carb diet.

Endeavor to purchase your bacon locally, without artificial additives, and don't burn it while cooking. It usually contains zero carbs; however, check the label and maintain a strategic distance from bacon that is treated with sugar.

- **Jerky (usually zero)**

Jerky is meat that has been processed into smaller strips and dried. As long as it doesn't contain added sugar or artificial additives, jerky can be an ideal low-carb snack food.

It is important you note that a lot of the jerky available at many stores is highly processed and therefore unhealthy. Your best option is to make your own.

Depending on the type, if it's mainly meat plus seasoning, it ought to be near zero carbs.

Other examples of low-carb meats include;

Turkey

Buffalo

Venison

Seafood

Fish and different kinds of seafood are usually extraordinarily nutritious and healthy. They're exceptionally high in B12, iodine, and omega-3 fatty acids—all nutrients which numerous individuals don't get enough of. Like beef, a wide range of fish and seafood contains almost no carbs.

• **Salmon (zero)**

Salmon is a standout amongst the most popular sorts of fish among health-conscious people—for obviously good reasons. It's a fatty fish, which implies that it contains large measures of heart-healthy fats, particularly omega-3 fatty acids. Salmon is additionally packed with vitamin B12, iodine, and a good amount of vitamin D3. It contains zero carbs.

• **Trout (zero)**

Like salmon, trout is a fatty fish that is stacked with omega-3 fatty acids and other essential vitamins. It has zero carbs.

• **Sardines (zero)**

Sardines are small, oily fish that are, for the most part, eaten whole, including their bones. Sardines are among the most nutrient-filled foods on earth and contain pretty much every vitamin that your body needs. They contain zero carbs.

- **Shellfish (4-5% carbs)**

It's shameful that shellfish almost never makes it onto some individuals' everyday menus as they're one of the world's most nutritious food. They rank near organ meats in their nutrient concentration and are low in carbs. They usually contain four to five grams of carbs per 100 grams of shellfish.

Other Low-Carb Fish and Seafood

Shrimp

Catfish

Haddock

Lobster

Herring

Cod

Vegetables

Most vegetables contain low carbs. Leafy greens and cruciferous vegetables have unusually low amounts, and the more substantial part of their carbs comprise of fiber. Then again, starchy root vegetables like potatoes and sweet potatoes are high in carbs.

Broccoli (7%)

Broccoli is a delicious cruciferous vegetable that can be eaten both raw and cooked. It's rich in vitamin C, vitamin K, and fiber and contains strong anti-cancer plant compounds. It contains six grams of carbs per cup, or seven grams for every 100 grams.

Tomatoes (4%)

Tomatoes are fruits or berries that are typically eaten as vegetables. They're high in potassium and vitamin C. There are seven grams of carb in an average large tomato or four grams for every 100 grams.

Onions (9%)

Onions are among the most delicious plants on earth and add incredible flavor to your meals. They're high in fiber, cancer prevention agents, and different inflammatory compounds. There are nine grams of carbs for every 100 grams.

Brussels Sprouts (7%)

Brussels grows exceptionally nutritious vegetables, closely related with broccoli and kale. They're high in vitamins C and K and contain various valuable plant compounds. There are about six grams of carbs for every half cup, or seven grams for every 100 grams.

Cauliflower (5%)

Cauliflower is a delicious and flexible vegetable that can be utilized to make different intriguing dishes in your kitchen. It's high in folate, vitamin C, and vitamin K. It contains five grams of carbs for each cup and five grams for every 100 grams.

Kale (10%)

Kale is a favorite vegetable among health-conscious people, offering various medical advantages.

It's stacked with fiber, vitamins C and K, and also carotene cancer prevention agents. It contains seven grams of carbs per cup, or 10 grams for every 100 grams.

Eggplant (6%)

Eggplant is another organic product that is generally devoured as a vegetable. It has many exciting uses and is high in fiber. It contains five grams of carbs cup, or six grams for every 100 grams.

Cucumber (4%)

Cucumber is a common vegetable with a gentle flavor. It is generally comprised of water, with a little measure of vitamin K. It contains two grams of carbs for every half cup, or four grams for every 100 grams.

Bell Peppers (6%)

Bell peppers are well known natural

products/vegetables with an unmistakable and fulfilling taste. They're high in fiber, vitamin C, and carotene cancer prevention agents. They contains nine grams of carbs for every cup, or six grams for every 100 grams.

Asparagus (2%)

Asparagus is a very delicious spring vegetable. It's high in fiber, vitamin C, folate, vitamin K, and carotene cancer prevention agents. Also, it's high in protein, contrasted with general vegetables. It contains three grams of carbs for every cup, or two grams for every 100 grams.

Green Beans (7%)

Green beans are legumes, yet they're usually eaten similarly as vegetables. Calorie by calorie, they're, to a significant degree, high in numerous nutrients, including vitamin C, protein, fiber, vitamin K, magnesium, and potassium. They contain eight grams of carbs for every cup, or seven grams for every 100 grams.

Mushrooms (3%)

Even though they're not plants, edible mushrooms are regularly grouped as vegetables. They contain decent measures of potassium and are highly concentrated in some B vitamins. They contain three grams of carbs for every glass, and three grams for every 100 grams (white mushrooms).

Other Low-Carb Vegetables

Celery

Spinach

Zucchini

Swiss chard

Cabbage

Except for starchy root vegetables, almost all vegetables have low-carb content. That is the reason you can eat a whole lot of them without going beyond your carb limit.

Fruits

Even though fruits are generally believed to be healthy, this is a bit controversial for those on a low-carb diet.

That is because most fruits will, in general, be high in carbs, as opposed to vegetables.

Depending on what amount of carbs you are planning to eat, you may need to confine your fruit intake to one to two pieces per day. However, this is not the case for fatty fruits like olives or avocados. Low-sugar fruits, for example, strawberries, are another excellent choice.

Avocado (8.5%)

The avocado is quite a unique kind of fruit. Rather than being high in carbs, it contains solid fats. Avocados are, to a significant degree, high in fiber and potassium and contain proper amounts of different nutrients.

When taking a look at the carb numbers below, remember that a large portion, or about at least 78 percent of the carbs in avocado, are fiber. Hence, they contain little or almost no digestible net carbs. They contain 13 grams of carbs for every cup, or 8.5 grams per 100 grams.

Olives (6%)

The olive is another nutritious and delicious high-fat fruit. It's high in iron and copper and contains a good amount of vitamin E. It contains about two grams of carbs for every ounce, or six grams for every 100 grams.

Strawberries (8%)

Strawberries are among the least carb-heavy and most nutrient-filled fruits you can eat. They're high in vitamin C, manganese, and different cancer prevention agents. They contain about 11 grams of carbs for every cup, or eight grams for every 100 grams.

Grapefruit (11%)

Grapefruits are citrus fruits that are very similar to oranges. They're high in carotene antioxidants and vitamin C. They contain about

There are 13 grams of carbs in half of a grapefruit, or 11 grams for every 100 grams.

Apricots (11%)

The apricot is an extraordinarily tasty fruit.

Every apricot contains few carbohydrates, plus a lot of potassium and vitamin. Two apricots contain about two grams of carbs, or there are 11 grams for every 100 grams.

Other Low-Carb Fruits

Lemons

Kiwis

Oranges

Nuts and Seeds

Nuts and seeds are exceptionally prominent on low-carb diets. They will, in general, be low in carbs, yet high in fat, fiber, protein, and different micro vitamins. Nuts are frequently eaten as snacks, while seeds are utilized for adding crunch to recipes and salads. Also, nut and seed flours—for example, coconut flour, almond flour, and flaxseed—are regularly used to make low-carb loaves of bread and other prepared meals.

Almonds (22%)

Almonds are unimaginably delicious and

crunchy. They're full of fiber and vitamin E and are one of the world's ideal sources of magnesium, a mineral that the vast majority don't get enough of. Additionally, almonds are fantastically satisfying and have been proven to improve weight loss in some research. They contain six grams of grams for every ounce, or 22 grams for every 100 grams.

Walnuts (14%)

The walnut is another delicious sort of nut. It contains different nutrients and is exceptionally high in alpha-linolenic acid (ALA), a kind of omega-3 fatty acid. Walnuts contain four grams of carbs for every ounce, or 14 grams for every 100 grams.

Peanuts (16%)

Peanuts are, in fact, legumes, yet will, in general, be prepared and consumed the same way as nuts.

They're high in magnesium, fiber, vitamin E, and other essential vitamins and minerals.

Chia Seeds (44%)

Chia seeds are, as of now, among the world's most well-known health foods. They're loaded with numerous essential vitamins and can be utilized in different low-carb-friendly menus.

Also, they're one of the most powerful sources of dietary fiber on the planet.

When taking a look at the carb numbers below, remember that about 86 percent of the carbs in chia seeds are fiber. Hence, they contain few digestible net carbs. They contain about 12 grams of carbs for every ounce, or 44 grams for every 100 grams.

Other Low-Carb Nuts and Seeds

Hazelnuts

Macadamia nuts

Cashews

Coconuts

Pistachios

Flaxseeds

Pumpkin seeds

Sunflower seeds

Dairy

If you're the type of person who tolerates dairy, then full-fat dairy products are great low-carb foods. In any case, make sure to peruse the label and abstain from anything with extra/added sugar.

Cheese (1.3%)

Cheese is a delicious low-carb food and can be eaten both raw and as an ingredient for preparing other meals. Furthermore, it goes exceptionally well with meat, for example, over a bun-less burger.

Cheese is profoundly nutritious. A single thick cut contains a comparative measure of nutrients to a whole glass of milk. It contains 0.4 grams of carbs per cup, or 1.3 grams per 100 grams (cheddar).

Heavy Cream (3%)

Heavy cream contains few carbs and little protein; however, it's high in dairy fat.

A few people on a low-carb diet add it in their coffee or use it in recipes. A bowl of berries with a decent amount of whipped cream can be a sweet low-carb dessert. It contains one gram of carb for every ounce, or three grams for every 100 grams.

Full-Fat Yogurt (5%)

Full-fat yogurt is incredibly healthy, containing a significant number of the same nutrients as whole milk.

On account of its live cultures, yogurt is likewise loaded with helpful probiotic bacteria. It contains 11 grams of carbs for each eight-ounce container, or five grams for every 100 grams.

Greek Yogurt (4%)

Greek yogurt, sometimes called strained yogurt, is highly different from regular yogurt. It's high in numerous helpful nutrients, particularly protein. It contains six grams of carbs for each six-ounce cup, or four grams for every 100 grams.

Fats and Oil

Numerous healthy fats and oils are adequate on a low-carb, genuine food-based diet.

Be that as it may, stay away from refined vegetable oils like corn oil or soybean as these are exceptionally unhealthy when consumed excessively.

- **Margarine/Butter (zero)**

Margarine, which was once demonized for its high saturated fat, has been making a rebound. You should go with grass-fed margarine since it's higher in specific nutrients. It contains zero carbs.

- **Extra Virgin Olive Oil (zero)**

Extra virgin olive oil is one of the most beneficial fats. It's a major ingredient in the heart-healthy Mediterranean diet, stacked with amazing cancer prevention agents and anti-inflammatory compounds. It contains zero carbs.

- **Coconut Oil (zero)**

Coconut oil is an excellent and healthy fat

stuffed with medium-chain fatty acids that have powerful, helpful benefits for your digestion. These fatty acids have been proven to diminish hunger, support fat burning, and help individuals lose tummy fat. It contains zero carbs.

Other Examples of Low-Carb-Friendly Fats include:

Tallow

Avocado Oil

Lard

Beverages

Most beverages without sugar are superbly satisfactory on a low-carb diet. Remember that fruit juices are high in sugar and carbs and ought to be avoided.

• **Water (zero)**

Water ought to be your go-to drink, regardless of whatever the rest of your diet looks like. It contains zero carbs.

- **Coffee (zero)**

Coffee is healthy and one of the largest sources of dietary antioxidants. Also, coffee consumers have been shown to live more and have a lower risk of some severe ailments, including type 2 diabetes, Parkinson's disease, and Alzheimer's. It contains zero carbs.

- **Tea (zero)**

Tea, particularly green tea, has been examined thoroughly and proven to have different noteworthy medical advantages. It might even slightly support the burning of fat. It contains zero carbs.

- **Club Soda/Carbonated Water (zero)**

Club soda is fundamentally water with added carbon dioxide. It's completely satisfactory as long as it has no sugar. Check the label to ensure it is sugar-free. It contains zero carbs.

Herbs and Condiments

There is a great variety of delicious spices, herbs, and condiments. Most of them contain very low carbs but contain powerful nutritional content and help add flavor to your meal. Some of the notable examples include salt, pepper, ginger, mustard, garlic, cinnamon, and oregano.

3.2 Benefits of having a shopping list.

Many times, we think we have a good grasp of grocery shopping such that we can head over to the store with an imaginary store in our heads. However, having a shopping list has its advantages. Beyond saving you time and money, it also makes you shop healthier and smarter. When we go to the store without planning, impulse buying is bound to happen, leading to us sometimes buying some unhealthy food items, or even completely forgetting to buy some of the things we need.

Here are a few reasons why you should have a shopping list:

Saves you time: Whenever we shop for groceries, we often spend money on impulse buying. Rather than filling your cart with all kinds of tempting and flashy items, a shopping list helps you stick with only the needed food items. When you don't fall for the temptation of buying all sorts of things, you will be saving more money.

Helps with meal planning: A shopping list assists in meal planning. When you sit down to write a list, you get to think and plan for what you need for the whole week. Beyond just buying essential food items, you also get to research interesting recipes and come up with new meal ideas. This benefit makes writing a shopping list more interesting and shopping much more fun.

Reduces food waste: Many times, a good portion of the food items that we buy go to waste. This is because often our eyes are bigger than our stomach when we purchase food items like fresh fruits and vegetables. These food items are highly perishable which means they'll get discarded once they go bad. When you have a shopping list, you can confidently buy the right quantities of food that you can eat without having so much going to waste.

Chapter 4: Simple and Easy Recipes to Start (7-Day Meal Plan)

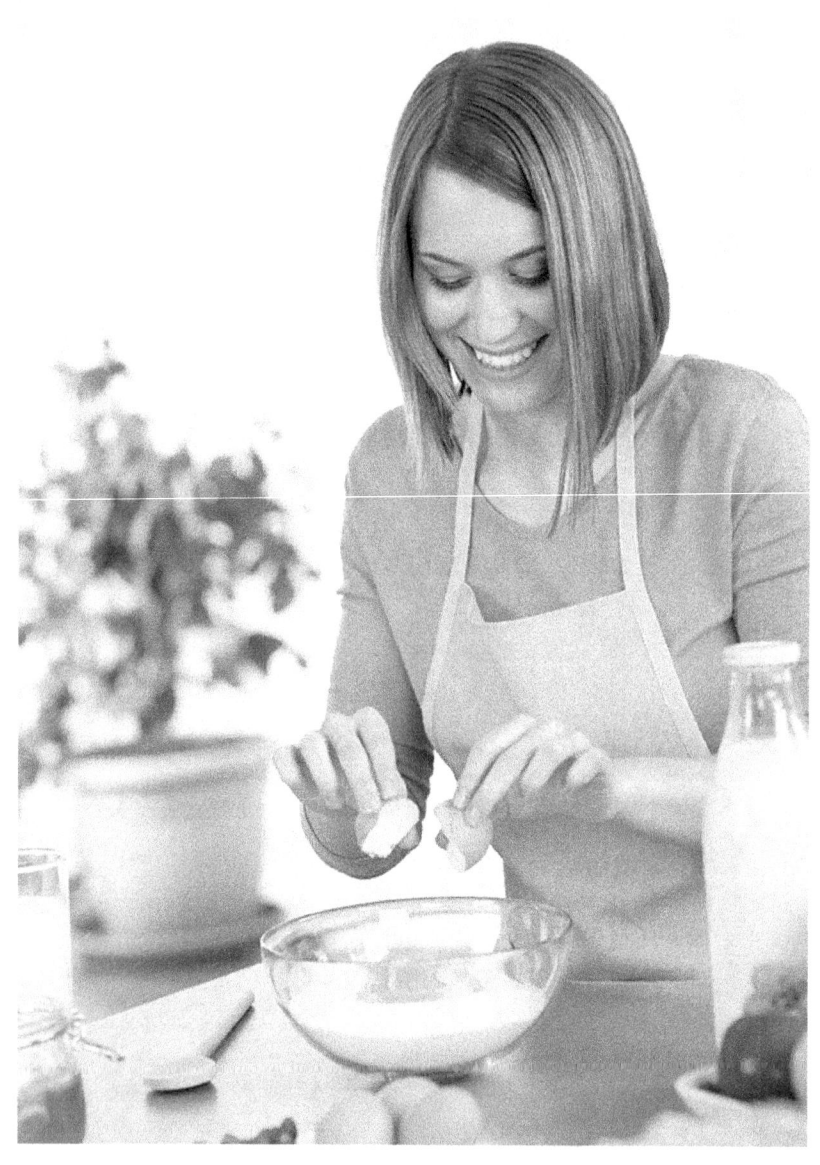

Chapter 4: Simple and Easy Recipes to Start (7- Day Meal Plan)

4.1 This section briefly discusses recipes you can eat while on the keto diet so that beginners will not be overwhelmed. They are recipes that are simple and easy to make that you can eat for a whole week.

4.2

Beyond the fact that these recipes are good for your health. There are other benefits that they bring along. Some of these benefits include:

- Easy to prepare: As opposed to popular thinking that preparing keto diet recipes are difficult to make, keto diet recipes are easy to prepare. All it takes is good planning.
- Flexibility: There's room for experimentation, revisions and customization in preparing these recipes.
- Delicious: These recipes are made using

tasty ingredients that will leave you wanting more and more.
- Look good: Keto recipes don't have to look terrible, they are in fact very appealing.
- Not expensive: Going on the keto diet is not expensive. Many of the recipes can be prepared at home thereby saving you extra cash that would have been spent eating out.

4.3

Here's a simple seven-day meal plan for you to follow. Don't forget that the point of the diet is to consume a whole lot of fat, low carbs, and a moderate amount of protein. Ways to prepare some of these recipes are included in later chapters. However, you can use the internet and find out how to cook any of the recipes mentioned here that are not explained in the book.

DAY 1

Breakfast: Cilantro and avocado with

scrambled egg lettuce wrap

Snack: Grilled chicken with olive oil dressing with kale salad

Lunch: Chicken-avocado lettuce wraps

Snack: Bell pepper with guacamole

Dinner: Cauliflower rice with steak

DAY 2

Breakfast: Baked egg in an avocado cup

Snack: Cold cut turkey roll-ups or sliced cheese

Lunch: Tuna salad and some green salad

Snack: Macadamia nuts

Dinner: Broccoli or Chinese beef

DAY 3

Breakfast: Full-fat Greek yogurt topped with chia seeds and crushed walnuts

Snack: Turkey jerky (specifically look for the type that has no sugar)

Lunch: Cauliflower fried rice

Snack: Sliced cheese

Dinner: Sautéed mushroom with roast beef and zucchini

DAY 4

Breakfast: Blackberry protein shake with almond butter with kale

Snack: Bacon deviled eggs

Lunch: Chicken tenders made using almond flour on a bed of greens with goat cheese and cucumbers

Snack: Zucchini parmesan chips

Dinner: Grilled shrimp topped with lemon butter sauce and some asparagus

DAY 5

Breakfast: Fried eggs and bacon with a side of greens

Snack: Celery sticks dipped in almond butter

Lunch: Grass-fed burger in a lettuce "bun" with avocado and a side salad

Snack: Half cup of coconut chips

Dinner: Meatloaf served on a bed of watercress salad

DAY 6

Breakfast: Feta cheese and spinach omelet

Snack: Bacon-wrapped asparagus

Lunch: Chicken wings with celery sticks

Snack: Cocoa coconut milk smoothie

Dinner: Bone broth recipe

DAY 7

Breakfast: Full-fat Greek yogurt with pumpkin seeds and coconut chips

Snack: Peanut butter fat bombs

Lunch: Chicken salad wraps

Snack: Cheese crisp

Dinner: Grilled salmon and a side of cauliflower rice

Your Quick-Start Action Step:

Carefully draft out your shopping list of things you'll need to get started on the diet. It doesn't have to be bulky, just ensure it contains enough items to successfully get you started.

Chapter 5:
The Recipes

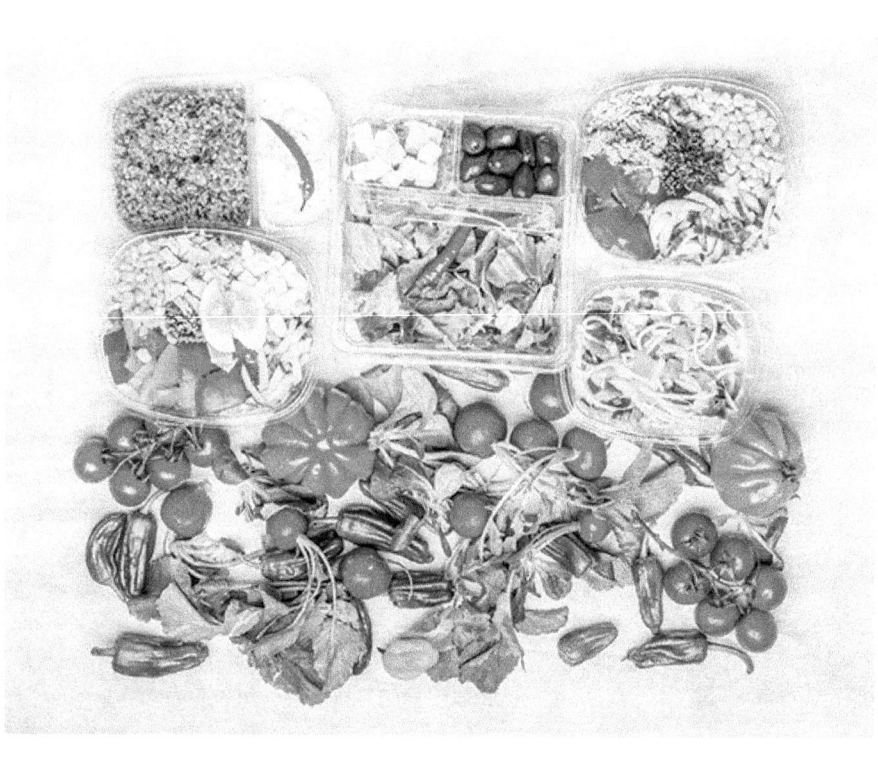

Chapter 5: The Recipes

5.1 The next few chapters are about some of the recipes you can take on the keto diet. These recipes are not just low in carb, they are equally delicious and pleasing to the eye. Going on the keto diet does not equate to eating unappealing meals. Feel free to experiment in your kitchen, just ensure you don't exceed your carb limit.

5.2 When you initially start your diet, it is normal to experience some difficulty; however, you must determine to never give up.
Having to eat only about 20 to 30 carbs can be challenging, especially at the start. Determination is what it takes.
Your body will equally show that there's changes in what you eat, that is what the "keto flu is all about." There'll be many days of weakness and being fatigued, it's all normal. Eventually, your body will adjust to it.

5.3 Your calorie intake is an important part of what determines weight loss or gain, and that is the reason why you must watch it. For many individuals, by just reducing the carb intake, however, if you intend to have a healthy lifestyle you need to keep up with the diet.

You don't have to use the recipes here alone, you can do further research on more keto-friendly recipes and try them out while on your diet. All it takes is proper planning. Plan, plan and plan again.

Your Quick Start Action Step:

Scan through the recipes in the next set of chapters to get a general idea on how to plan into your routine and schedule.

Chapter 6: Breakfast

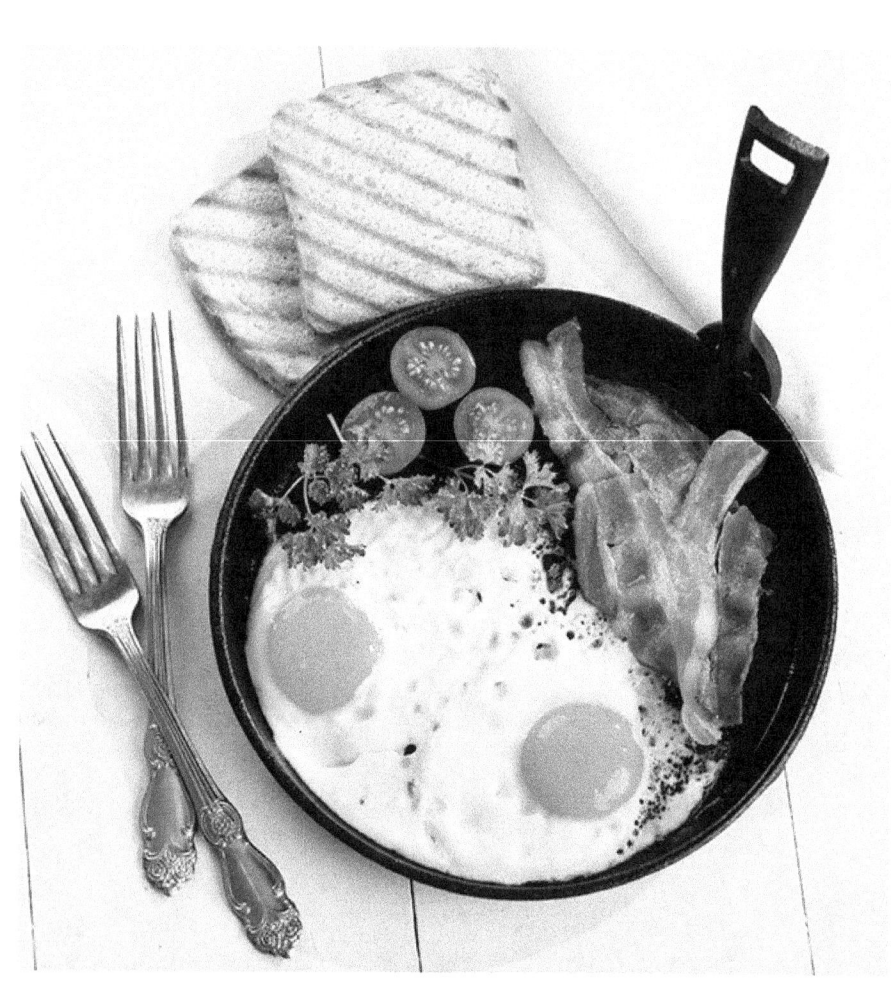

Chapter 6: Breakfast

Keto Frittata With Fresh Spinach

This dish is more than beautiful; it is delicious yet easy to prepare. Spinach, sausage, eggs or bacon, and vegetables all contribute to making this a glorious meal both for the eyes and the tummy. It's a gold star on the keto diet list.

Ingredients

5 oz. diced bacon or chorizo

Eight eggs

Salt and pepper

2 tablespoons butter, for frying

8 oz. fresh spinach

5 oz. shredded cheese

1 cup heavy whipping cream

Instructions

- Preheat the oven until it gets to about

350°F (175°C).
- Then fry the bacon in margarine at medium-high heat until it's crispy. Add the spinach to the bacon and keep stirring until it wilts. Remove the pan from the heat and keep it aside.
- Whisk the eggs and the cream and pour into an oiled baking dish (9×9 inches) or in separate ramekins.
- Add the bacon, cheese, and spinach on top of it and place it right in the middle of the oven.
- Bake for 25 or 30 minutes or till it is set in the middle and golden brown on top.
- You could try it with shredded red or green cabbage with homemade dressing. Have a delicious breakfast.

Nutritional information:

Net carbs: 2% (4 g)

Fiber: 1 g

Fat: 81% (59 g)

Protein: 16% (27 g)

Kcal: 661

Lemon-Cashew Smoothie

The cashew milk with the heavy cream combines to create a tasty smoothie that is good enough to refresh and still makes for a great breakfast or snack. By adding a few ice cubes, it will be like enjoying a rich citrus sorbet rather than a healthy breakfast. A couple of leaves of fresh mint will also enhance the fresh flavor.

Ingredients

1 cup unsweetened cashew milk

1/4 cup heavy (whipping) cream

1/4 cup freshly squeezed lemon juice

1 scoop plain protein powder

1 tablespoon coconut oil

1 teaspoon sweetener

Instructions

- Put the heavy cream, cashew milk, lemon

juice, protein powder, coconut oil, and sweetener in a blender and blend until smooth.
- Pour into a glass and serve immediately.
- Almond milk or coconut milk are also excellent choices instead of cashew milk if you prefer those products. Each type of milk adds a slightly different flavor to the smoothie, so try them all to get the right combination for your palate.

Nutritional information:

Net carbs: 7% (15 g)

Fiber: 4 g

Fat: 80% (45 g)

Protein: 13% (29 g)

Kcal: 503

Nut Medley Granola

Homemade granola is incredibly versatile. It is a treat to have ready-made for breakfast, snacks, and as a healthy topping for a creamy cup of Greek yogurt. The mix and amount of nuts in this recipe create a wonderful keto macro; however, you can add or omit different ingredients as you wish. Don't add dried fruits though, because they are very high in carbs.

Ingredients

2 cups shredded unsweetened coconut

1 cup sliced almonds

1 cup raw sunflower seeds

1/2 cup raw pumpkin seeds

1/2 cup walnuts

1/2 cup melted coconut oil

10 drops liquid stevia

1 teaspoon ground cinnamon

1/2 teaspoon ground nutmeg

Instructions

- Preheat the oven to 250°F. Line two baking sheets with parchment paper and

set aside.
- Toss together the almonds, shredded coconut, sunflower seeds, pumpkin seeds, and walnuts in a large bowl until mixed.
- In a small bowl, stir the coconut oil, cinnamon, stevia, and nutmeg until blended.
- Pour the coconut oil mixture and the nut mixture together and blend using your hands until the nuts are well coated.
- Transfer the granola mixture to baking sheets and spread it out evenly.
- Bake the granola. Ensure you stir every 10 to 15 minutes until the mixture turns golden brown and is crunchy.
- Move the granola to a large bowl and allow it to cool, tossing frequently to break up the large pieces. You can store the granola in containers in the refrigerator or freezer for up to one month.

Nutritional information:

Net carbs: 10% (10 g)

Fiber: 6 g

Fat: 80% (38 g)

Protein: 10% (10 g)

Kcal: 391

Bacon-Artichoke Omelet

Omelets are not just for breakfast, and this vegetable- and bacon-packed beauty is hearty enough for a light dinner. If you add a nice mixed green salad to the plate, you won't go over your carbs because the combination with the omelet should still be an excellent keto macro. If you have leftovers, try them cold the next day for a snack or lunch.

Ingredients

6 eggs, beaten

2 tablespoons heavy (whipping) cream

8 bacon slices, cooked and chopped

1 tablespoon olive oil

1/4 cup chopped onion

1/2 cup chopped artichoke hearts (canned, packed in water)

Sea salt

Freshly ground black pepper

Instructions

- In a small bowl, whisk the eggs, bacon and heavy cream until well blended, and set aside.
- Place a large skillet over medium-high heat and add olive oil.
- Sauté the onion until tender, about 3 minutes.
- Pour the egg mixture into the skillet. Swirl it for 1 minute.
- Cook the omelet. Lift the edges using a spatula to let the uncooked egg flow underneath for 2 minutes.
- Sprinkle the artichoke hearts on top and flip the omelet. Cook for 4 minutes

more, until the egg is firm. Flip the omelet over again, so the artichoke hearts are on top.

- Remove from the heat, cut the omelet into quarters, and season with salt and black pepper. Transfer the omelet to plates and serve.

Nutritional information:

Net carbs: 5% (5 g)

Fiber: 2 g

Fat: 80% (39 g)

Protein: 15% (17 g)

Kcal: 435

Keto Blt With Cloud Bread

Whenever you say "BLT," the atmosphere begins to change! You can have it alongside the great fluffy cloud bread, popularly called "oopsie bread." It's a grain-free and gluten-free bread. A taste will leave you wanting more!

Ingredients

1 pinch salt

1/2 tablespoon baking powder

4 1/4 oz. cream cheese

1/2 tablespoons ground psyllium husk powder

1/4 cream of tartar (optional)

3 eggs

Toppings

2 oz. lettuce

1 tomato, thinly sliced

8 tablespoons mayonnaise

5 oz. bacon

Fresh basil (optional)

Cloud bread

Instructions

- Preheat the oven until 30ºF (15ºC).
- Then separate the eggs. Separate the egg whites from the yolks and put them in

separate bowls.
- Whip the egg whites together with salt (with cream of tartar, if you want to use any) until they are very stiff. You can do this using a handheld electric mixer. You should be able to turn over the bowl without the egg whites moving.
- Add some cream cheese to the egg yolks and mix. To make the oopsie more bread-like, add some baking powder (optionally, you can also add psyllium seed husk).
- Gently fold all the egg whites into the egg yolk mixture in such a way that there is air in the egg whites.
- Put about 8 oopsie bread pieces on a paper-lined baking tray.
- Bake in the middle of the oven for up to 25 minutes until they look golden.

Building the BLT

- Fry the bacon using a skillet at medium-high heat until it's crispy.
- Turn the oopsie bread piece upside down.
- Spread one or two tablespoons of mayonnaise on each piece.
- Place the lettuce, fried slices of bacon,

tomato, and some finely chopped fresh basil in layers in the middle of each bread.

Nutritional information:

Net carbs: 3% (4 g)

Fiber: 1 g

Fat: 88% (48 g)

Protein: 9% (11 g)

Kcal: 498

Peanut Butter Cup Smoothie

If you're a lover of the famous candy featuring chocolate and peanut butter, then you will enjoy the same flavor blend for breakfast or even as a filling snack. If you want a more chocolatey taste, then add a teaspoon of good-quality cocoa powder and a couple of drops of liquid stevia. These additions will not add any fat, protein, or carbs to the smoothie

Ingredients

1 cup water

3/4 cup coconut cream

1 scoop chocolate protein powder

2 tablespoons natural peanut butter

2 ice cubes

Instructions

- Put the coconut cream, water, protein powder, peanut butter, and ice in a blender and blend until smooth.
- Pour into 2 glasses and serve immediately.

Nutritional Information

Net carbs: 2% (4 g)

Fiber: 5 g

Fat: 70% (40 g)

Protein: 20% (30 g)

Kcal: 486

Keto Mexican Scrambled Eggs

You can spice up your breakfast with this sumptuous keto egg meal. Tomatoes, jalapeños, and scallions can be used to enhance the scrambled eggs with the right quantity of zing; this is a great way to start your day.

Ingredients

1 scallion

6 eggs

Salt and pepper

1 tomato, finely chopped

2 tablespoons butter, for frying

3 oz. shredded cheese

2 pickled jalapeños, finely chopped

Instructions

- Start by chopping the scallions, tomatoes, and jalapeños. Fry them in butter for about 3 minutes on medium heat.

- Break the eggs and pour into a pan. Scramble for about 2 minutes. Add some cheese and seasonings.
- Serve with crisp lettuce, avocado, and dressing to make it more colorful.

Nutritional information:

Net carbs: 3% (2 g)

Fiber: 1 g

Fat: 72% (18 g)

Protein: 24% (14 g)

Kcal: 221

Classic Bacon And Eggs

This is one of the best keto breakfast ever. Enhance your bacon and egg meal with this style. You can eat as many eggs as you need to feel satisfied.

Ingredient

5 oz. bacon, in slices

8 eggs

Fresh parsley (optional)

Cherry tomatoes (optional)

Instruction

- Fry the bacon using a pan at medium-high heat until it is crispy. Remove the fried bacon and set it aside on a plate and leave the rendered fat inside the pan.
- Use the same pan you used in frying the bacon to fry the eggs. Place the pan over medium heat and beat your egg into the bacon fats (alternatively, you can break the eggs into a cup and gently pour into the pan to avoid splattering hot grease).
- Cook the eggs whichever way you like. For eggs cooked over easy, turn the eggs over after some minutes, then cook for one more minute. For sunny-side up, allow the eggs to fry on one side and cover the pan to ensure they get cooked on top.
- You should cut the cherry tomatoes and

fry at the same time.
- Add salt and pepper to taste.

Nutritional information:

Net carbs: 2% (1 g)

Fiber: 0 g

Fat: 75% (22 g)

Protein: 23% (15 g)

Kcal: 272

Keto Mushroom Omelet

If you need an easy and quick way to start your day, then this mushroom omelet is for you. It is super healthy and only takes a few minutes to prepare. You can enjoy this meal for breakfast; it also passes for lunch and dinner.

Ingredients

3 mushrooms

3 eggs

Salt and pepper

1 oz. butter, for frying

1/5 yellow onion

1 oz. shredded cheese

Instructions

- Beat the egg into a bowl and mix with pepper and a pinch of salt. Use a fork to whisk the egg until it is smooth and frothy.
- Add some salt and spices.
- Melt some margarine into a frying pan. When it melts, add the egg mixture. By the time the omelet starts to cook and get firm, but still has some raw egg, sprinkle mushrooms, cheese, and onion on top.
- Use a spatula to ease around the edges of the omelet gently and fold it over in equal halves. Once the color begins to change to golden brown beneath, remove the pan from the heat and set the omelet on a plate.

- Serve the omelet alongside a crispy green salad.

Nutritional information:

Net carbs: 3% (4 g)

Fiber: 1 g

Fat: 77% (43 g)

Protein: 20% (25 g)

Kcal: 510

Iced Tea

Cold and refreshing iced tea. It is thirst quenching; hence, you won't notice the absence of sugar. Have the feel of summer all year round with this great beverage.

Ingredient

1 tea bag

1 cup ice cubes

2 cups cold water

Your choice of flavorings, e.g., fresh mint or sliced lemon

Instructions

- Add the tea to half of the cold water and flavoring in a mug and refrigerate for about 1 to 2 hours.
- Remove the tea bag as well as the flavoring. You can replace the flavoring if you want.
- Add the other half of the cold water and serve with plenty of ice cubes.

Nutritional information:

Net carbs: 0% (0 g)

Fiber: 0 g

Fat: 0% (0 g)

Protein: 0% (0 g)

Kcal: 0

Chapter 7:
Soups and Salads

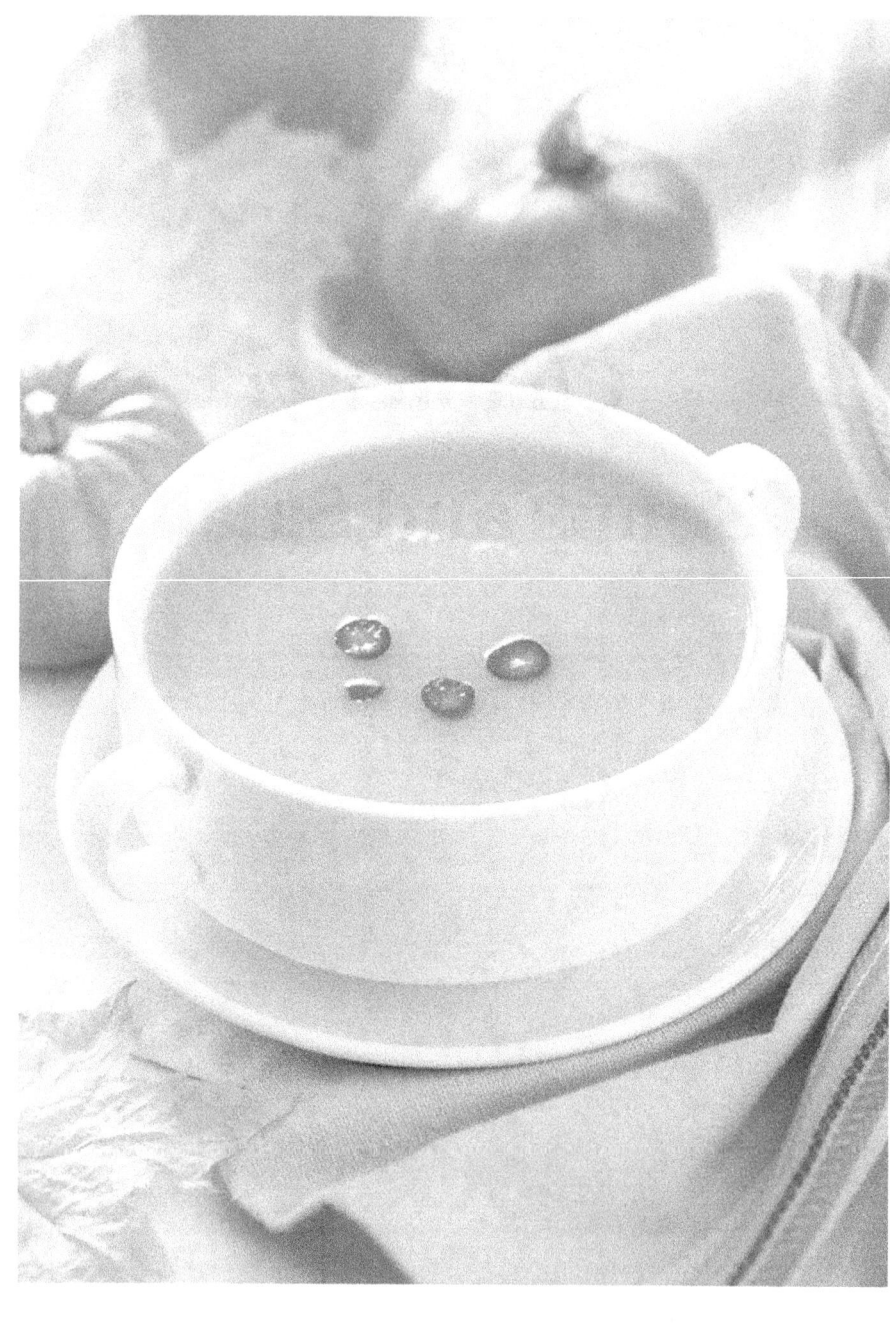

Chapter 7: Soups and Salads

7.1 Soups and Salads
Low-Carb Pumpkin Soup

This is a great soup to eat in the evening.

Ingredients

2 garlic cloves

2 shallots

10 oz. pumpkins

2 tablespoons olive oil

8 oz. butter

1 tablespoon salt

1/2 tablespoon ground black pepper

10 oz. rutabaga

2 cups vegetable stock

1/2 lime, the juice

Toppings

4 tablespoons pumpkin seeds, preferably roasted

3/4 cup mayonnaise

Instructions

- Start by heating the oven until it gets to about 400ºF (200ºC). Peel the pumpkin and the rutabaga and cut the flesh into

small cubes. Cut the shallot into wedges and peel the garlic as well.
- Put all of them into a baking dish. Add some salt, pepper, and olive oil.
- Roast them in the oven for about 25 to 30 minutes. Alternatively, you could also try frying using medium-high heat with a large pan until both the pumpkin and the turnip get soft.
- Put the roasted veggies into a pot. Add vegetable stock or water and leave it to boil. Leave it to simmer for some minutes after which you can remove it from the stove.
- Add some butter, divided into cubes. Using a hand blender, mix the soup. Add salt and pepper to taste, juice, and herbs.
- You can have the soup served with mayonnaise, parmesan croutons, or roasted pumpkin seeds.
- Try to make it spicy. Cumin, chili, and some other spices can be used in making this soup. Add some freshly grated ginger a few minutes before serving; it will bring

a new kind of twist to the flavor.

Nutritional information:

Net carbs: 6% (14 g)

Fiber: 3 g

Fat: 91% (88 g)

Protein: 3% (6 g)

Kcal: 865

Homemade Chicken Stock

Chicken has a great flavor. You can use it in making stews and sauces. Make a great stew using the chicken stock, and you have a nutrient-filled meal.

Ingredients

1 chicken

1 leek

1 carrot

1 bay leaf

1 yellow onion

1 tablespoon white peppercorn

1/2 cup dry white wine (optional)

2 tablespoons olive oil

2 garlic cloves

Salt

6 cups water

Instructions

- Peel and grate your vegetables into smaller pieces.
- Use olive oil in a big pot to brown the vegetables; you should use an enamel cast pot. Brown them until they have a beautiful color.
- Divide the chicken into equal halves. Pour some spices and water into the pot, cover the pot, reduce the heat, and allow it to simmer for up to 2 hours.
- Remove the chicken and extract the bones until you have just meat left. If you love the chicken skin crispy, then you should spread the chicken skin on an oven sheet lined with clean parchment paper.
- Add some spices to taste, then bake using the oven at about 400°F (200°C) for at least 15 minutes, or better still, until they are crispy.
- Break the chicken bones into smaller pieces and pour back into the pot. Allow

it to simmer for 3 more hours.
- Filter your stock using a fine strainer and pour the stock into the pot. Reduce it to about half or more (depending on how rich you want your stock). The stock is not meant to be overcooked; allow it to simmer using medium-low heat. Add some salt towards the end.
- You can have this stored in your refrigerator for 2 to 3 days or freeze it in smaller containers for at least 3 months. It is awesome to use it as a natural flavor enhancer in sauces, pots, and soups.

Nutritional information:

Net carbs: 1% (0.5 g)

Fiber: 0 g

Fat: 81% (13 g)

Protein: 18% (7 g)

Kcal: 145

Blt Salad

The servings of this salad are quite small, but the combination of ingredients packs an intense flavor burst. Using bacon fat in the dressing rather than olive oil adds much more flavor to this already mouthwatering salad. Bacon fat will keep in a sealed container in the refrigerator for up to one week, so save it for other recipes whenever you cook bacon.

Ingredients

2 tablespoons melted bacon fat

2 tablespoons red wine vinegar

Freshly ground black pepper

4 cups shredded lettuce

1 tomato, chopped

6 bacon slices, cooked and chopped

2 hardboiled eggs, chopped

1 tablespoon roasted unsalted sunflower seeds

1 teaspoon toasted sesame seeds

1 cooked chicken breast, sliced (optional)

Instructions

- Use a medium bowl to whisk the vinegar and bacon fat until emulsified. Season with black pepper.
- Add the tomato and lettuce to the bowl and toss the vegetables with the dressing.
- Divide the salad into 4 plates and top each with equal amounts of egg, bacon,

sesame seeds, sunflower seeds, and chicken (if using). Serve.

Nutritional information:

Net carbs: 7% (4 g)

Fiber: 2 g

Fat: 76% (18 g)

Protein: 17% (1 g)

Kcal: 228

Cauliflower-Cheddar Soup

Cauliflower is a popular vegetable that can be eaten on the keto diet in many recipes, like this creamy soup. Cauliflower is a good source of manganese, vitamins C and K, and omega-3 fatty acids which improve brain function, help support digestion, and promote a healthy heart. You should choose a snow-white head of cauliflower with crisp green leaves and no brown spots.

Ingredients

1/2 sweet onion, chopped

1 cup heavy (whipping) cream

1 head cauliflower, chopped

1/4 cup butter

4 cups herbed chicken stock

1/2 teaspoon ground nutmeg

Sea salt

Freshly ground black pepper

1 cup shredded cheddar cheese

Instructions

- Place a large pot over medium heat and add butter.
- Sauté the onion and cauliflower until tender and lightly browned, about 10 minutes.
- Add the nutmeg and chicken stock to the pot and bring the liquid to a boil.
- Then reduce the heat and allow it to simmer until the vegetables are soft.
- Remove the pot from the heat and stir in the heavy cream. Purée the soup with a food processor or an immersion blender until smooth.
- Salt and pepper the soup. Serve topped with the cheddar cheese.

Nutritional information:

Net carbs: 9% (4 g)

Fiber: 2 g

Fat: 81% (21 g)

Protein: 12% (8 g)

Kcal: 227

Wild Mushroom Soup

The warm mushroom keto soup is a delight. It is particularly creamy and smooth.

Ingredients

5 oz. portabella mushrooms

5 oz. shiitake mushrooms

5 oz. oyster mushrooms

4 oz. butter

1 garlic clove

1 cup heavy whipping cream

1 tablespoon white wine vinegar

3 cups water

1/2 cup thyme

1/2 lb. celery root

1 vegetable bouillon cube or chicken bouillon cube

Fresh parsley (optional)

Instructions

- Wash, trim, and cut the mushrooms and celery root. Peel the onion and garlic and

finely chop them.
- Sauté the chopped vegetables in margarine using medium heat in a heavy-bottomed saucepan until it turns brown. Reserve some mushroom for serving.
- Add vinegar, thyme, bouillon cube, and water and allow it to boil. Reduce the heat and allow to simmer for up to 15 minutes or until the celery is soft enough.
- Add some cream and puree using an immersion blender until you achieve the fineness you want. Serve it with some pieces of sautéed mushroom and finely chopped parsley.
- Feel free to try out some other mushroom types like porcini, chanterelles, and white-buttoned mushrooms.

Nutritional information:

Net carbs: 10% (11 g)

Fiber: 3 g

Fat: 85% (45 g)

Protein: 5% (6 g)

Kcal: 468

Green Gazpacho

This is a great chilled keto soup that you can try during hot summer months. It's simply a blend of all the ingredients into a drinkable soup.

Ingredients

1/2 cup diced celery stalks

1/2 cup presoaked drained cashew nuts

1/2 cup peeled, seeded and sliced cucumber

1/2 cup watercress leaves

5 oz. Romaine lettuce (5 large crisp leaves)

1 garlic clove

1/4 cup extra virgin oil

1 cup chicken broth

1 tablespoon fine salt

Instruction

- Put all ingredients into a blender and keep blending until smooth and creamy. You can serve and enjoy.
- You can soak the cashews in salty water for about 3 hours to minimize the phytic acid content in them, thereby aiding the digestion.

Nutritional information:

Net carbs: 11% (9 g)

Fiber: 2 g
Fat: 82% (29 g)
Protein: 6% (5 g)
Kcal: 311

Spicy Almond And Seed Mix

The spicy almond and seed mix with a blend of cumin are awesome as a snack or even as topping for soups and salads. It is guaranteed to be completely free of additives.

Ingredients

1 cup almonds

2 tablespoons olive oil or coconut oil

1/3 cup sunflower seeds

1/3 cup pumpkin seeds

1 tablespoon ground and crushed fennel or cumin seeds

1/2 tablespoon salt

1 tablespoon chili paste

Instructions

- Preheat the oil in a large frying pan, then add the chili.
- Add the almonds and seeds, then stir thoroughly.

- Sauté for some minutes and add salt. You must note that almonds and seeds are sensitive to heat, so ensure the oil is hot enough to allow the spice flavors to develop. However, ensure the almonds and seeds don't get burnt.
- Allow to cool, then store in a glass container.
- You can serve it as a snack or as a topping with cauliflower soup or as a crispy flavor enhancer.

Nutritional information:

Net carbs: 6% (2 g)

Fiber: 3 g

Fat: 81% (15 g)

Protein: 13% (6 g)

Kcal: 166

Greek Egg And Lemon Soup With Chicken

If you want something creamy without using real cream, try out this Greek recipe, "avgolemono." It is very easy to prepare. All you need is chicken, eggs, cauliflower, and butter.

Ingredients

2 chicken bouillon cubes

1 lb. boneless chicken thighs

1 bay leaf

4 cups water

3/4 lb. cauliflower

4 eggs

1/3 lb. butter

2 tablespoons fresh thyme or fresh parsley

1 lemon—zest and juice

Salt and ground black pepper

Instructions

- Slice the chicken thigh into thin pieces, place it in a saucepan, add some cold water, and boil. Add bay leaf and some bouillon cubes.
- Reduce the heat to medium and allow it to simmer for about 10 minutes or until the chicken is thoroughly cooked.
- Remove the bay leaf and meat from the heat and don't allow the broth to get cold.
- Grate the cauliflower until it resembles rice and put it in the saucepan.
- Increase the heat, add some butter, and

boil for a few minutes. Break the eggs into a bowl and add lemon juice.
- Add salt and pepper to taste.
- Reduce the heat and then add the eggs. Stir continuously and allow to simmer for a few minutes until the soup becomes slightly thick, but don't boil; it will likely curdle.
- Add the chicken back to the soup. Serve with lemon zest and some finely chopped thyme or parsley.

  You can reheat the soup using medium heat until it simmers. But be careful so it doesn't boil. It will still be delicious, but you sure don't want the curdled look.

  Alternatively, you can skip steps 1 and 2 and warm up the poultry in the broth in step 6.

Nutritional information:

Net carbs: 3% (5 g)

Fiber: 2 g

Fat: 79% (54 g)

Protein: 17% (27 g)

Kcal: 620

Chapter 8: Snacks and Side Dishes

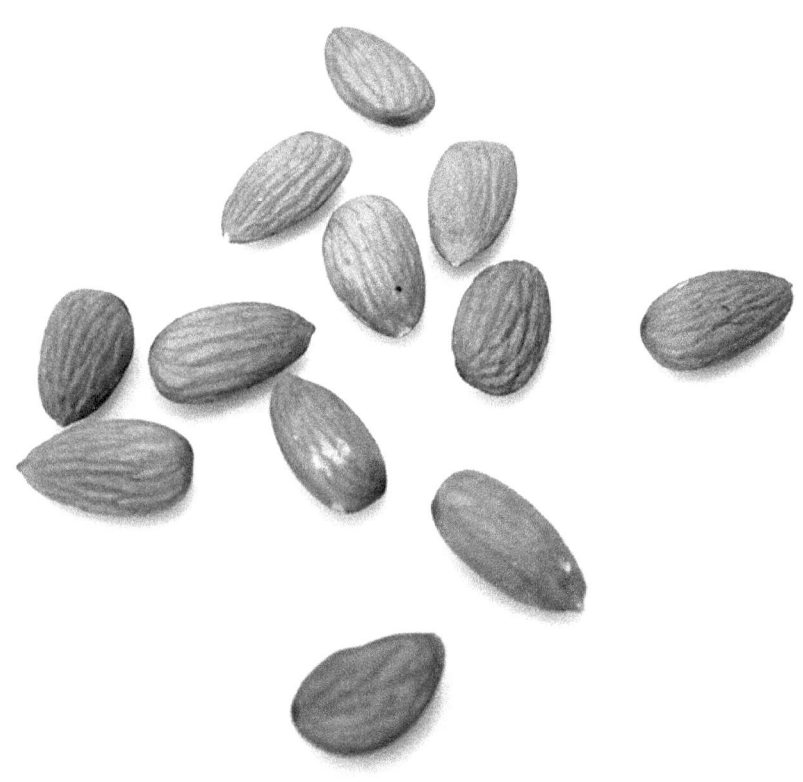

Chapter 8: Snacks and Side Dishes

Low-Carb Cauliflower Rice

If you're missing rice, then here is the perfect low-carb substitute. Cauliflower rice is awesome eaten with Asian dishes and is a good replacement for pasta or couscous. It's neutral and finely textured.

Ingredients

3 oz. butter or coconut oil

25 oz. cauliflower

1/2 tablespoon salt

1/2 tablespoon turmeric (optional)

Instructions

- Use a grater to shred the cauliflower head.
- Melt margarine or coconut oil in a skillet. Add the cauliflower and cook using

medium heat for about 5 to 10 minutes or until the riced cauliflower softens.
- Salt it, and optionally, add some turmeric while frying.
- You can cook the grated cauliflower using the microwave. Place it in a glass plate and cover it with a plastic wrap. Microwave it for about 5 to 6 minutes. Mix the butter or coconut oil and allow it to melt.
- You can make your cauliflower rice "au naturel"—skip the turmeric. Or you can use a different herb to spice it up like curry, herb salt, or paprika powder.

Nutritional information:

Net carbs: 11% (6 g)

Fiber: 4 g

Fat: 82% (19 g)

Protein: 7% (4 g)

Kcal: 208

Creamed Green Cabbage

It's soft and easy. It also goes with everything. This creamy keto dish is so good, you'll be tempted to make a whole lot for you to enjoy all week.

Ingredients

25 oz. green cabbage

2 oz. butter

1/2 cup fresh, finely chopped parsley

1 1/4 cups whipping heavy cream

1/2 zest lemon

Salt and pepper

Instructions

- You should start by shredding the cabbage by slicing thinly with a sharp knife or with a food processor.
- Melt the margarine in a frying pan on medium-high heat. Add cabbage and sauté for some minutes until it gets soft

and the color changes to golden around the edges.
- Add plenty of whipping cream and allow the cabbage simmer until the cream reduces. Reduce the heat towards the end.
- Add pepper and salt to taste.
- Add some parsley and lemon zest just before serving. If you want to reduce your daily dairy consumption, you can switch the heavy whipping cream with coconut cream or coconut oil.

Nutritional information:

Net carbs: 9% (9 g)

Fiber: 5 g

Fat: 87% (38 g)

Protein: 5% (5 g)

Kcal: 401

Crab Salad-Stuffed Avocado

Depending on the size of your avocados, this decadent dish could be a filling snack or a light lunch. It's perfectly acceptable to use frozen crab if fresh is not available, but be careful to look for real crab meat rather than cheaper imitation products. If using frozen crab, thaw it completely and squeeze out any extra liquid so that your salad isn't soggy.

Ingredients

1 avocado, peeled, halved lengthwise, and pitted

1/2 teaspoon freshly squeezed lemon juice

4 1/2 ounces Dungeness crabmeat

1/2 cup cream cheese

1/4 cup chopped red bell pepper

1/4 cup chopped, peeled English cucumber

1/2 scallion, chopped

1 teaspoon chopped cilantro

Pinch sea salt

Freshly ground black pepper

Instructions

- Brush the cut edges of the avocado with the lemon juice and set the halves aside on a plate.
- In a medium bowl, stir the crabmeat, cream cheese, red pepper, cucumber, scallion, cilantro, salt, and pepper until well mixed.
- Split the crab mixture between the avocado halves and store them, covered with plastic wrap, in the refrigerator until you're ready to serve them (up to 2 days).

Nutritional information:

Net carbs: 10% (10 g)

Fiber: 5 g

Fat: 70% (31 g)

Protein: 20% (19 g)

Kcal: 389

Turkey Rissoles

Chicken is often the first choice for poultry in most home kitchens, but turkey is fabulous tasting, inexpensive, and very healthy. Turkey is low in fat and high in protein. Make sure some of your other recipe ingredients are high in fat so your keto macro is perfect. Turkey can help boost your immunity because it contains an amino acid called tryptophan, which supports the immune system.

Ingredients

1-pound ground turkey

1 scallion, green and white parts, finely chopped

1 teaspoon minced garlic

Pinch sea salt

Pinch freshly ground black pepper

1 cup ground almonds

2 tablespoons olive oil

Instructions

- Preheat the oven to 350°F (175°C). Line a baking sheet with aluminum foil and set

it aside.
- In a medium bowl, mix the turkey, scallion, garlic, salt, and pepper until well combined.
- Mold the turkey mixture into 8 patties and flatten them out.
- Place the ground almonds in a shallow bowl and dredge the turkey patties in the ground almonds to coat.
- Place a large skillet over medium heat and add the olive oil.
- Brown the turkey patties on both sides, about 10 minutes in total.
- Transfer the patties to the baking sheet. Bake them until cooked through, flipping them once, about 15 minutes in total.
- Make the whole recipe from start to finish and place the cooled turkey patties in sealed plastic bags and store them in the refrigerator for up to 3 days or the freezer for up to 1 month.
- Take them out of the freezer and thaw for a quick dinner or snack or reheat them right from the refrigerator.

Nutritional information:

Net carbs: 10% (10 g)

Fiber: 5 g

Fat: 70% (31 g)

Protein: 20% (19 g)

Kcal: 389

Roasted Pork Loin With Grainy Mustard Sauce

This is a delicious sauce; you might have to double the amount you make because eating it by the spoonful as a snack is a real treat. It is also stellar with barbecued beef tenderloin or a perfectly roasted lamb rack.

Ingredients

3 tablespoons grainy mustard, such as Pommery

1 (2-pound) boneless pork loin roast

Freshly ground black pepper

3 tablespoons olive oil

Sea salt

1 1/2 cups heavy (whipping) cream

Instructions

- Preheat the oven to 375°F (175°C).
- Season the pork roast all over with sea salt and pepper.
- Place a large skillet over medium-high heat and add the olive oil.
- Roast until all sides turn brown in the skillet. This will take about 6 minutes in total, then place the roast in a baking dish.
- Roast until a meat thermometer put in the thickest part of the roast reads 155°F (72°C), about 1 hour.
- When there are about 15 minutes of roasting time left, place a small saucepan over medium heat and add the heavy cream and mustard.
- Stir the sauce until it simmers, then reduce the heat to low. Simmer the sauce

until it is very rich and thick, about 5 minutes.

- Remove the pan from the heat and set aside. Let the pork cool for 10 minutes before you slice and serve with the sauce.

Nutritional information:

Net carbs: 5% (2 g)

Fiber: 0 g

Fat: 70% (29 g)

Protein: 25% (25 g)

Kcal: 368

Portobella Mushroom Pizza

Mozzarella is prepared using a method that spins the milk from the cheese and then cuts it. The method is called pasta filata.

Mozzarella is a great choice for the keto diet. It is high in fat (65 percent), contains about 32 percent protein, and has only three percent carbs.

Ingredients

4 large Portobella mushrooms, stems removed

1/4 cup olive oil

1 teaspoon minced garlic

1 medium tomato, cut into 4 slices

2 teaspoons chopped fresh basil

1 cup shredded mozzarella cheese

Instructions

- Start by preheating the oven to broil. Line a baking sheet with clean aluminum foil and set it aside.
- Using a small bowl, toss the mushroom caps with the olive oil until well coated.
- Use your fingertips to rub the oil in. Avoid breaking the mushrooms.
- Place the mushrooms on the baking sheet, gill-side down, and broil the mushrooms until they are tender on the tops, about 2 minutes.
- Turn the mushrooms over and broil 1

minute more.

- Take out the baking sheet and spread the garlic over each mushroom, top each with a tomato slice, sprinkle with the basil, and also top with the cheese.
Broil the mushrooms till the cheese is melted and bubbly, about 1 minute, and serve.

These pizzas pack a lot of flavors, so you'll need an assertive main course to share the plate with them. Some wonderful options could include Bacon-Wrapped Beef Tenderloin or Sirloin with Blue Cheese Compound Butter. These juicy mushrooms make a tempting snack, as well.

Nutritional information:

Net carbs: 10% (7 g)

Fiber: 3 g

Fat: 71% (20 g)

Protein: 19% (14 g)

Kcal: 251

Low-Carb Eggplant Hash With Eggs

Are you missing the old potato hash? If so, then you should try this one out! A delicious and easy to make keto-friendly meal that the entire household should love.

Ingredients

4 eggs

2 eggplants

2 tablespoons olive oil

1 yellow onion

2 tablespoons butter

8 oz. halloumi cheese or any other cheese that can be fried

1/2 tablespoon Worcestershire sauce (optional)

Instructions

- Peel and finely chop the onion.

- Dice the halloumi cheese and eggplant into 1/2-inch cubes.

  Fry the onion in oil using medium heat until it gets soft. Add eggplant and halloumi and fry until it all turns golden brown.
- Add salt and pepper to taste.
- Fry the eggs using whatever style you wish in another pan. You can optionally serve with some drops Worcestershire sauce.

  You should buy small or medium-sized eggplants; they are usually better than the larger ones in terms of flavor.

Nutritional information:

Net carbs: 11% (11 g)

Fiber: 8 g

Fat: 69% (31 g)

Protein: 20% (20 g)

Kcal: 423

Low-Carb Onion Rings

This is one of the easiest recipes you can make. It's simply onion made into rings. They can be eaten alongside chicken, burgers, or anything grilled. It's so simple, yet so delicious.

Ingredients

1 jumbo onion

1 cup almond flour

1 egg

1 tablespoon olive oil

1 tablespoon garlic powder

½ cup grated parmesan cheese

½ tablespoon powder or paprika powder

1 pinch of salt

Instructions

- Start by preheating the oven until it reaches about 400°F (200C).
- Peel and slice the onion into rings that are about 1/5 inch thick.

- Mix all ingredients in a bowl while you beat and whisk the egg in a separate bowl.
- Dip the onion rings into the egg batter and dip in a flour mix as well, one at a time.
- You can put the rings of onions in a baking sheet covered with parchment paper.
- Spray oil on the rings and bake using an oven for about 15 to 20 minutes. If you're using the broiler, ensure you monitor them closely; they're ready once the color changes to golden brown and they are crisp.

Nutritional information:

Net carbs: 7% (5 g)

Fiber: 1 g

Fat: 74% (26 g)

Protcin: 19% (15 g)

Kcal: 323

Spicy Keto Roasted Nuts

They're spicy, crunchy, salty, and snacky. These nuts will have your guests asking for more.

Ingredients

8 oz. almonds, walnuts, or pecans.

1 tablespoon coconut oil or olive oil

1 tablespoon chili powder or paprika powder

1 tablespoon ground cumin

1 tablespoon salt

Instructions

- Add all ingredients in a medium frying pan and mix thoroughly. Cook using medium heat until the almonds have been warmed.
- Allow it to cool. Serve as a snack, or eat alongside a drink.
- Store at room temperature in a container with a lid.

You don't necessarily have to use almonds; you can use other types of nuts, e.g., pecans.

Nutritional information:

Net carbs: 3% (2 g)

Fiber: 4 g

Fat: 92% (29 g)

Protein: 5% (4 g)

Kcal: 281

Keto Cheese Puffs

They're simple, crunchy, and crispy.

Ingredients

5 1/3 oz. Brie cheese (preferably President Brie)

Instructions

- Cut the rind off the Brie cheese and cut it into small 1/2-inch cubes. Ensure you remove the white edge.

- Put some pieces of the brie cheese on a paper. Put on a plate and use a microwave oven to bake at full power for 1 to 2 minutes. You should observe it to ensure it doesn't get burnt. Don't make too many at a time.
- Allow to cool before serving. You can season it with whatever spices you want.

Nutritional information:

Net carbs: 1% (0.2 g)

Fiber: 0 g

Fat: 75% (14 g)

Protein: 25% (10 g)

Kcal: 167

Chapter 9:
Fish and Poultry

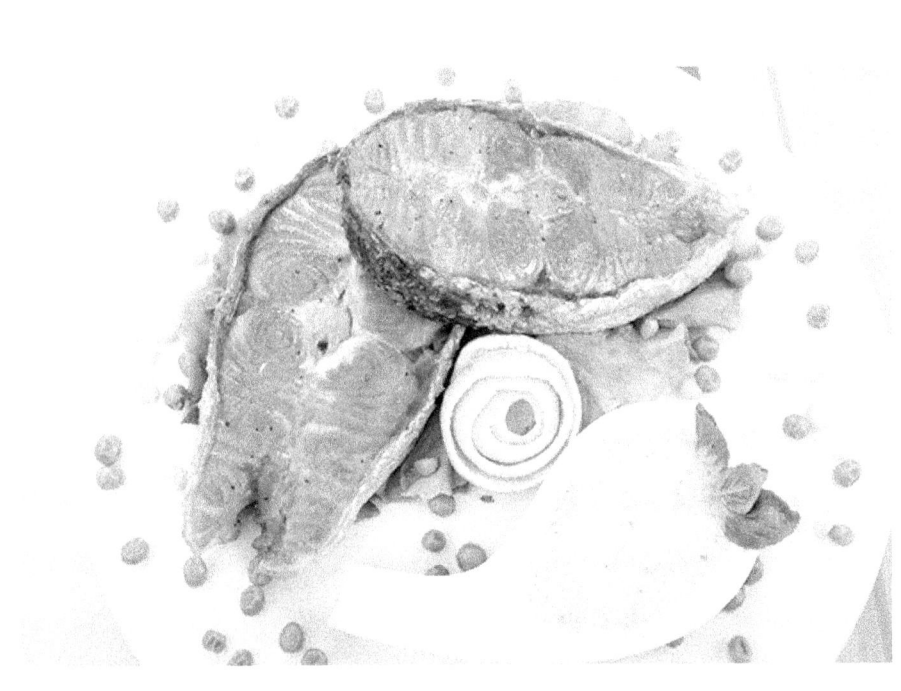

Chapter 9: Fish and Poultry

Keto Salmon With Pesto And Spinach

If you love both salmon and pesto, then this dish is for you.

Ingredients

1 tablespoon green or red pesto

25 oz. salmon

2 oz. grated parmesan cheese

1/6 oz. butter or olive oil

1 lb. fresh spinach

Instructions

- Start by heating the oven until it reaches about 400°F (2000c).
- Grease the baking dish with oil or about half of the butter.
- Add salt and pepper to the salmon fillets and put them in the prepared baking dish, skin-side down.
- Mix the pesto, mayonnaise, and

- parmesan cheese and spread on top of the salmon.
- Bake the mixture for about 15 to 20 minutes, or until the salmon easily flakes with a fork.
  Meanwhile, you should use the remaining oil or butter to sauté the spinach until it wilts. After 2 minutes, season with pepper and salt.
- You can serve along with the salmon that was baked in the oven.

Nutritional information:

Net carbs: 1% (3 g)

Fiber: 3 g

Fat: 79% (78 g)

Protein: 20% (45 g)

Kcal: 902

Keto Tuna Casserole

You can use this as a good replacement for

noodles. It's made with peppers, onions, celery, and can be prepared in about 30 minutes.

Ingredients

1 green bell pepper

2 oz. butter

5 1/3 oz. celery stalks

1 cup mayonnaise

4 oz. freshly shredded parmesan cheese

16 oz. tuna in drained olive oil

1 yellow onion

1 tablespoon chili flakes

Instructions

- Start by preheating the oven until it reaches 400°F (200°C). Finely chop the celery bell, pepper, and onion.
- Fry the chopped ingredients in margarine until it is relatively soft. Add salt and pepper to taste.
- Mix the chili flakes, mayonnaise,

parmesan cheese, and tuna in an oiled baking dish. Add some fried vegetables and stir.
- Allow to bake in the oven for about 15 to 20 minutes or until golden brown.

Nutritional information:

Net carbs: 2% (5 g)

Fiber: 3 g

Fat: 80% (83 g)

Protein: 18% (43 g)

Kcal: 953

Keto Baked Salmon With Butter And Lemon

Simply a great meal

Ingredients

2 lbs. salmon

1 tablespoon olive oil

Black ground pepper

1 lemon

7 oz. butter

Instructions

- Start by preheating the oven until it reaches 400°F (200°C).
- Put a little amount of olive oil in the large baking dish. Put the salmon in skin- side down. Add pepper and salt according to your taste.
- Slice the lemon into thin pieces and put it on top of the salmon. Use half of the butter to cover the salmon
- Place it on the middle rack of the oven and bake for at least 20 to 30 minutes, or until the salmon looks opaque and easily flakes with a fork.
- Put the remaining butter in a small saucepan and heat until it begins to bubble.
- Remove from the stove and allow to cool for a little while. Gently add some of the

lemon juice.
- You can serve the fish with any side dish you want with the lemon butter.
You can try adding lemon zest to your butter.

Nutritional information:

Net carbs: 0% (1 g)

Fiber: 0 g

Fat: 78% (49 g)

Protein: 22% (31 g)

Kcal: 573

Sweet And Sticky Chicken Wings

They have layers of aromas, textures, and flavors that will excite your senses. Crispy and juicy, savory and sweet at the same time. It brings back childhood memories of sticky fingers.

Ingredients

2 lbs. chicken wings

3/4 cup coconut aminos

1 1/2 tablespoon sea salt

1/4 tablespoon onion powder

1/4 tablespoon ground ginger

1/4 tablespoon garlic powder

1/4 tablespoon chili flakes

Instructions

- Start by preheating the oven until it reaches 450°F (230°C).
- Place the chicken wings on a rimmed baking sheet that has wire racks, thicker skin side facing up. The wire racks help enhance the cooking.
- Sprinkle some fine pink Himalayan sea salt or any other salt on the wings.
- Allow the wings to bake for about 45 minutes.
- Using medium heat, heat a medium-sized or large skillet and then add the

coconut aminos.
- You can now add the onion powder, garlic powder ginger powder, and some red pepper flakes if you want. Once the sauce begins to simmer, start stirring. Continue occasionally stirring while adjusting the heat accordingly to ensure a gentle simmer.
- Once you notice that the sauce has started thickening (when you stir it, it usually should take only a few seconds to rise and fill your spatula or spoon), you can reduce the heat while the wings finish cooking.
- Put the wings in a large heat-resistant bowl and pour the sauce on them. Serve after you have stirred to coat evenly.

Nutritional information:

Net carbs: 3% (10 g)

Fiber: 3 g

Fat: 5% (3 g)

Protein: 8% (4 g)

Kcal: 67

Keto Chicken And Cabbage Plate

This is an example of a keto dinner that is not complicated.

Ingredients

7 oz. fresh green cabbage

1 lb. rotisserie chicken

1/2 red onion

1/2 cup mayonnaise

1 tablespoon olive oil

Salt and pepper

Instructions

- Cut the cabbage with a sharp knife and place on a plate.
- Slice the onion into thin pieces and put it with the chicken on the same plate. Also add a good quantity of mayonnaise.

- Sprinkle some olive oil on the cabbage.
- Add some pepper and salt to taste.
  You can make use of leftover chicken rather than rotisserie chicken.

Nutritional information:

Net carbs: 3% (7 g)

Fiber: 3 g

Fat: 79% (91 g)

Protein: 19% (48 g)

Kcal: 1041

Simple Fish Curry

Curry is a sauce-based recipe originating in India and adopted by many cultures.

The ubiquitous spice mixture often contains a multitude of ingredients such as cumin, coriander, turmeric, ginger, cloves, paprika, and cinnamon. It's adapted so well to many cuisines because no matter the ingredients used—

vegetables, meats, fish, eggs, butter, or coconut—the spices bring the dish together beautifully.

Ingredients

2 tablespoons coconut oil

1 1/2 tablespoons grated fresh ginger

2 teaspoons minced garlic

1 tablespoon curry powder

1/2 teaspoon ground cumin

2 cups coconut milk

16 ounces firm white fish, cut into 1-inch chunks

1 cup shredded kale

2 tablespoons chopped cilantro

Instructions

- Place a large saucepan over medium heat and melt the coconut oil.
- Sauté the ginger and garlic until lightly browned, about 2 minutes.

- Stir the curry powder and cumin and sauté until very fragrant, about 2 minutes.
- Stir in the coconut milk and bring the liquid to a boil.
- Reduce the heat and allow it to simmer for about 5 minutes to infuse the milk with the spices.
- Add the fish and cook until the fish is cooked through about 10 minutes.
- Stir in the kale and cilantro and simmer until wilted, about 2 minutes, and serve.

Nutritional information:

Net carbs: 6% (5 g)

Fiber: 1 g

Fat: 70% (31 g)

Protein: 24% (26 g)

Kcal: 416

Pan-Seared Halibut With Citrus Butter

Sauce

Citrus fruits are delicious and are bursting with nutrients. Both lemons and oranges are excellent sources of vitamin C, which boosts the immune system and can help detoxify your body. The acid from citrus is a wonderful addition to most fish and seafood recipes.

Ingredients

4 (5-ounce) halibut fillets, each about 1-inch thick

Sea salt

Freshly ground black pepper

1/4 cup butter

2 teaspoons minced garlic

1 shallot, minced

3 tablespoons dry white wine

1 tablespoon freshly squeezed lemon juice

1 tablespoon freshly squeezed orange juice

2 teaspoons chopped fresh parsley

2 tablespoons olive oil

Instructions

- Dry the fish by patting with paper towels and then lightly season the fillets with salt and pepper. Set aside on a paper towel-lined plate.
- Place a small saucepan over medium heat and melt the butter.
- Sauté the garlic and shallot until tender, about 3 minutes.
- Whisk in the white wine, lemon juice, and orange juice and bring the sauce to a simmer. Cook until it thickens slightly, about 2 minutes.
- Remove the sauce from the heat and stir in the parsley; set aside.
- Place a large skillet over medium-high heat and add olive oil.
- Panfry the fish until lightly browned and just cooked through, turning over once, about 10 minutes in total.
- Serve the fish immediately with a spoonful of sauce for each.

Any firm white-fleshed fish will be delicious with this creamy sauce. Try haddock, tilapia, or sea bass.

Nutritional information:

Net carbs: 1% (2 g)

Fiber: 0 g

Fat: 70% (26 g)

Protein: 29% (22 g)

Kcal: 319

Roasted Salmon With Avocado Salsa

Simple, fresh salsa is often the best topping for a juicy piece of fish, and creamy avocados are a perfect choice for the base. Take the salsa ingredients out of the refrigerator an hour or so before serving the fish, so they come to room temperature.

The taste of the avocado will be much stronger than when this fruit is completely chilled. You can also grill the salmon for this recipe—this fish holds up well under higher heat and does not dry out.

Ingredients for the Salsa

1 avocado, peeled, pitted, and diced

1 scallion, white and green parts, chopped

1/2 cup halved cherry tomatoes

Juice of 1 lemon

Zest of 1 lemon

Ingredients for the Fish

1 teaspoon ground cumin

1/2 teaspoon ground coriander

1/2 teaspoon onion powder

1/4 teaspoon sea salt

Pinch freshly ground black pepper

Pinch cayenne pepper

4 (4-ounce) boneless, skinless salmon fillets

2 tablespoons olive oil

Instructions on how to make the Salsa

- In a small bowl, stir the avocado, scallion, tomatoes, lemon juice, and lemon zest until mixed and set aside.

Instructions on how to bake the Fish

- Preheat the oven to about 400°F (200°C). Line a baking sheet with clean aluminum foil and set aside.
- In a small bowl, stir the cumin, coriander, onion powder, salt, black pepper, and cayenne until well mixed.
- Rub the spice mix on the salmon fillets and place them on the baking sheet.
- Drizzle the fillets with the olive oil and roast the fish until just cooked through, about 15 minutes.
- Serve the salmon alongside the avocado salsa.

Nutritional information:

Net carbs: 5% (4 g)

Fiber: 3 g

Fat: 69% (26 g)

Protein: 26% (22 g)

Kcal: 320

Sole Asiago

Sole is a flatfish, which means both of its eyes are on one side of its head. It looks rather strange, but when filleted, it is delicious. Sole is not a threatened species, but it is overfished in some areas, so it is not as plentiful as it was in the past. This tender, delicate fish freezes very well; if you cannot find fresh fillets, frozen fillets will work, too.

Ingredients

4 (4-ounce) sole fillets

3/4 cup ground almonds

1/4 cup Asiago cheese

2 eggs, beaten

2 1/2 tablespoons melted coconut oil

Instructions

- Preheat the oven to 350°F (175°C). Line a baking sheet with clean parchment paper and set aside.
- Pat the fish dry with paper towels.
- Stir together the ground almonds and cheese in a small bowl.
- Place the bowl with the beaten eggs next to the almond mixture.
- Dredge a sole fillet in the beaten egg and then press the fish into the almond mixture, so it is completely coated. Place on the baking sheet and repeat until all the fillets are breaded
- Brush both sides of each piece of fish with the coconut oil.
- Bake the sole until it is cooked through, about 8 minutes in total.
- Serve immediately.

Nutritional information:

Net carbs: 5% (6 g)

Fiber: 3 g

Fat: 65% (31 g)

Protein: 30% (29 g)

Kcal: 406

Keto Fajita Chicken Casserole

It's made with great flavors. Perfect for weekends.

Ingredients

7 oz. cream cheese

1 rotisserie chicken

1/3 cup mayonnaise

1 yellow onion

1 red bell pepper

7 oz. shredded pepper

2 tablespoons Tex-Mex seasoning

Salt and pepper

Instructions

- Start by preheating the oven until it reaches 400°F (200°C).
- Cut the chicken into small pieces. Chop or grate the peppers and onions.
- Mix all the ingredients, leaving a third of cheese in an already greased baking dish.
- Add the remaining cheese and bake for about 15 to 20 minutes or until golden brown.
- You can serve with greens dressed in olive oil.

Nutritional information:

Net carbs: 3% (10 g)

Fiber: 3 g

Fat: 77% (98 g)

Protein: 20% (57 g)

Kcal: 1148

Chapter 10:
Pork and Beef

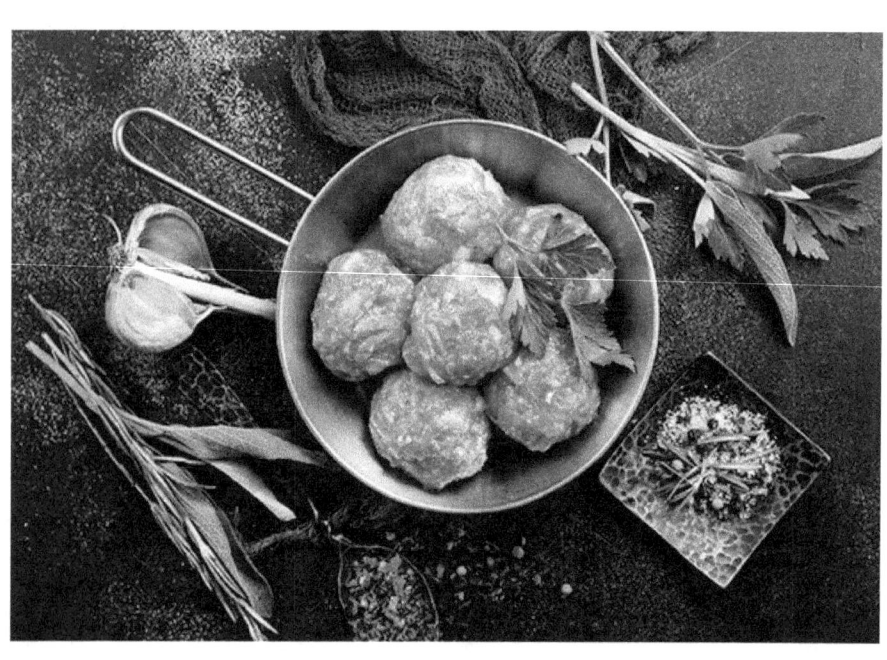

Chapter 10: Pork and Beef

Keto Pimiento Cheese Meatballs

They are simply delicious. They're good for both dinner and snacking.

Ingredients

Pimiento

Cheese

1/4 cup pimientos or pickled jalapeños

1/3 cup mayonnaise

1 pinch cayenne pepper

1 tablespoon Dijon mustard

1 egg

1 tablespoon chili powder or paprika powder

25 oz. ground beef

2 tablespoons butter, for frying

Salt and pepper

Instructions

- Mix all the ingredients in a large bowl and set aside for a few minutes.
- Add the egg and ground beef to the mixture. Mix properly using clean hands or a wooden spoon. Add salt and pepper to taste.
- Mold large meatballs and fry in a skillet with margarine or oil at medium-high heat until thoroughly cooked.
- You can serve with whatever side dish you desire, homemade mayonnaise, and maybe a green salad.

Nutritional information:

Net carbs: 1% (1 g)

Fiber: 1 g

Fat: 73% (53 g)

Protein: 26% (42 g)

Kcal: 660

Classic Keto Hamburger

This is delicious and can be eaten with keto buns.

Ingredients

5 oz. cooked bacon

1 3/4 lbs. ground beef

2 oz. shredded lettuce

8 tablespoons mayonnaise

1 red onion

1 oz. olive oil or margarine, for frying

1 tomato

Salt and pepper

Ingredients for the keto hamburger buns

5 tablespoons ground psyllium husk powder

1 1/4 cups almond flour

3 eggs

1 1/4 cups boiling water

3 tablespoons baking powder

1 tablespoon sesame seeds

3 egg whites

2 tablespoons cold vinegar or white wine

Instructions

- Heat the oven to 350°F (175°C)
- Begin the cooking by preparing the hamburger buns. Mix the dry ingredients in a dry bowl.
- Boil the water and add it, the egg whites, and the vinegar to the bowl while mixing with a hand mixer for up to 30 seconds. Don't overmix the dough; make it as smooth as Play-Doh.
- Use moist hands to mold the dough into pieces of bread, one per serving. Sprinkle some sesame seeds over it. Ensure you create some space on the baking sheet to accommodate the buns when they double in size.
- Put on the lower rack in the oven and bake for about 50 to 60 minutes. Once you hear a slight sound when you tap the

bottom of the buns, that's a sign that they are ready.

Preparing the hamburgers

While the bread is baking, you can prepare the condiments. Slice the onion and tomato thinly, shred the lettuce, and fry the bacon.

Mold the ground beef into single pieces of hamburger and grill or fry. Add some salt and pepper to taste when the hamburger is almost ready.

Cut the bread into halves and lavishly spread a good quantity of mayonnaise on both halves.

Make your hamburger the way you want it to taste.

Eat with coleslaw as a side for extra crunch.

Nutritional information:

Net carbs: 3% (6 g)

Fiber: 10 g

Fat: 76% (87 g)

Protein: 21% (54 g)

Kcal: 1067

Keto Ground Beans And Green Beans

This meal is a real wonder; it's affordable and simple to prepare. Perfect for dinner and yet fast food.

Ingredients

9 oz. fresh green beans

10 oz. ground beef

1/3 cup crème fraiche or mayonnaise (optional)

Salt and pepper

3 1/2 oz. margarine

Instructions

- Wash and trim the green beans.
- Heat a good amount of margarine with a frying pan that can hold both the green beans and the ground beef.
- Use high heat to brown the ground beef until it's almost ready and then add salt

and pepper.
- Reduce the heat, add extra margarine, and fry the beans for about 5 minutes, using the same pan. You should stir the ground beef very often.
- Add salt and pepper to the beans. You can then serve the remaining margarine and add some crème fraiche or mayonnaise if you need more fat for satisfaction.
- You can make this meal using other low-carb veggies like asparagus, spinach, zucchini, or broccoli. Use your choice of spices to add more flavor to the vegetables, meat, and dip.

Nutritional information:

Net carbs: 3% (5 g)

Fiber: 3 g

Fat: 78% (60 g)

Protein: 19% (32 g)

Kcal: 694

Chapter 11: Desserts and Treats

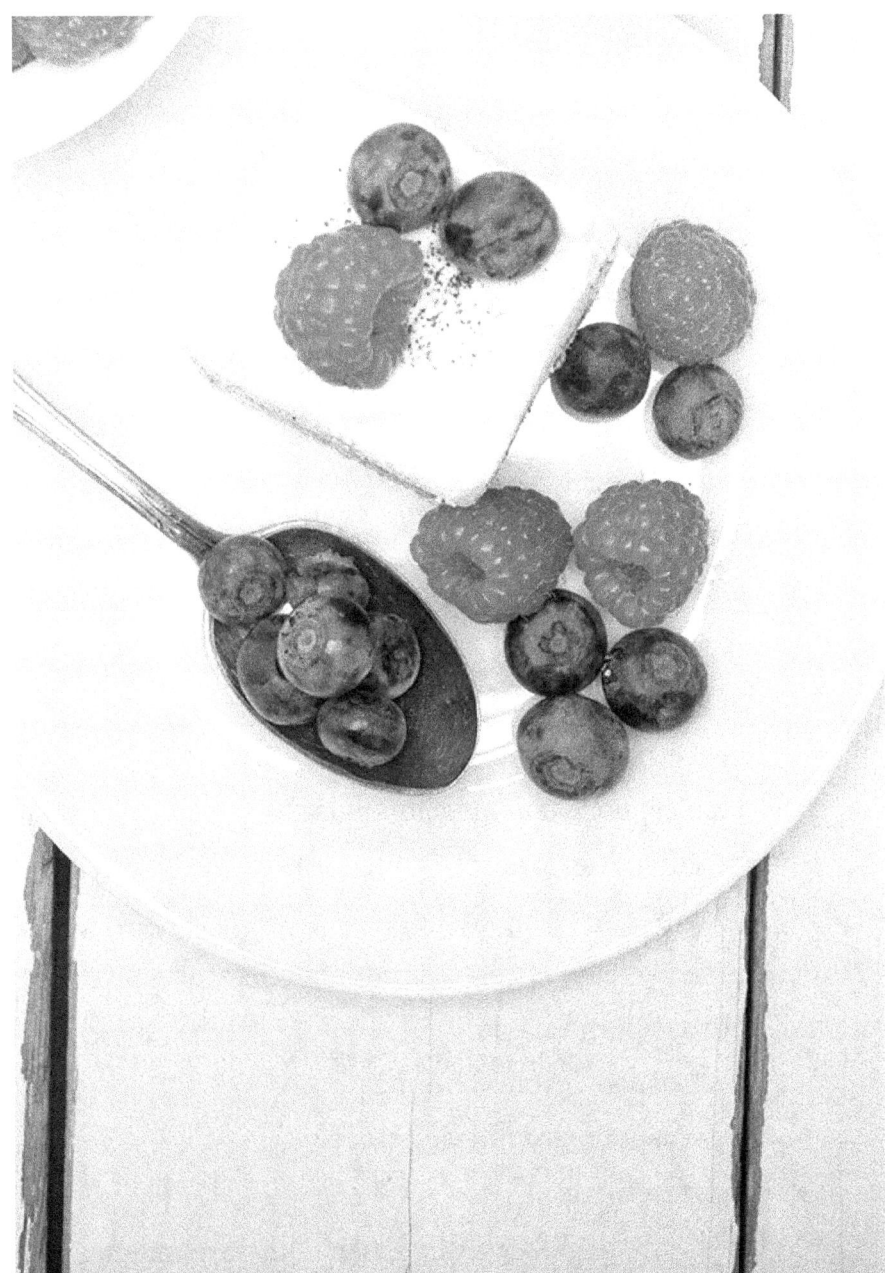

Chapter 11: Desserts and Treats

Pumpkin Spice Fat Bombs

Pumpkin is a natural choice for desserts, especially those that also include warm spices reminiscent of holiday pumpkin pie. Like its vegetable counterpart, carrots, the bright orange flesh of pumpkin indicates it is a stellar source of beta-carotene.

Pumpkin is also very high in vitamins A and C as well as potassium, making this pretty ingredient perfect for flushing toxins from your body and fighting cancer.

Ingredients

3 tablespoons chopped almonds

1/2 cup butter, at room temperature

1/3 cup pure pumpkin purée

1/2 cup cream cheese, at room temperature

4 drops liquid stevia

1/4 teaspoon ground nutmeg

1/2 teaspoon ground cinnamon

Instructions

- Line an 8-by-8-inch pan with parchment

paper and set aside.
- In a small bowl, whisk the butter and cream cheese together until very smooth.
- Add the pumpkin purée and whisk until blended.
- Stir in the almonds, cinnamon, stevia, and nutmeg.
- Spoon the pumpkin mixture into the pan. Use a spatula or the back of a spoon to spread it evenly in the pan, then place in the freezer for about 1 hour.
- Cut into 16 pieces and store the fat bombs in a tightly sealed container in the freezer until ready to serve.

Nutritional information:

Net carbs: 5% (1 g)

Fiber: 0 g

Fat: 90% (9 g)

Protein: 5% (1 g)

Kcal: 87

Chocolate-Coconut Treats

Chocolate and coconut are a flawless combination often found in candy bars and many desserts. If you want a more elegant presentation, omit the coconut in step 3 and roll the semi-hardened chocolate mixture into balls instead of spreading in a pan. Then roll the balls in the shredded coconut and place the treats in the freezer to firm up completely.

Ingredients

¼ cup unsweetened cocoa powder

1/3 Cup coconut oil

Pinch sea salt

1/4 cup shredded unsweetened coconut

4 drops liquid stevia coconut

Instructions

- Line a 6-by-6-inch baking dish with parchment paper and set aside.
- In a small saucepan over low heat, stir together the coconut oil, cocoa, stevia, and salt for about 3 minutes.
- Stir in the coconut and press the mixture into the baking dish.
- Place the baking dish in the refrigerator

until the mixture is hard, about 30 minutes.
- Cut into 16 pieces and store the treats in an airtight container in a cool place.
  For a more finished look, you can spoon the hot mixture into candy molds instead of a baking dish. Pop the molds in the refrigerator for 30 minutes or until firm and pop the treats out into a container.

Nutritional information:

Net carbs: 6% (1 g)

Fiber: 0 g

Fat: 88% (5 g)

Protein: 6% (1 g)

Kcal: 43

Almond Butter Fudge

Fudge should be smooth and dense with no grittiness or graininess. Since you won't be using granulated sugar for this treat, the chances of getting the wrong texture are greatly reduced. Almond butter is a stellar source of protein, vitamin E, iron, manganese, and fiber. If you are not a fan of this nut butter, peanut butter or cashew butter would also be delicious and creates the same tempting results.

Ingredients

1 cup coconut oil, at room temperature

1/4 cup heavy (whipping) cream

1 cup almond butter

10 drops liquid stevia

Pinch sea salt

Instructions

- Line a 6-by-6-inch baking dish with parchment paper and set aside.
- In a medium bowl, whisk together the heavy cream, almond butter, coconut oil, stevia, and salt until very smooth.
- Spoon the mixture into the baking dish and smooth the top with a spatula.
- Place the dish in the refrigerator until the fudge is firm, about 2 hours.
- Cut into 36 pieces and store the fudge in an airtight container in the freezer for up to 2 weeks.

Nutritional information:

Net carbs: 5% (3 g)

Fiber: 1 g

Fat: 90% (22 g)

Protein: 5% (3 g)

Kcal: 204

Nutty Shortbread Cookies

Traditional shortbread has very few ingredients and is intensely buttery, slightly crumbly, and not too sweet. The nuts used here in place of flour create the desired texture and add a complex, pleasing flavor. These cookies will continue to cook on the baking sheets after you eat them out of the oven, so don't forget to transfer them to wire racks quickly to avoid over-browning.

Ingredients

1/2 cup butter, at room temperature, plus additional for greasing baking sheet
1 1/2 cups almond flour
1/2 cup granulated sweetener

1/2 cup ground hazelnuts

1 teaspoon alcohol-free pure vanilla extract

Pinch sea salt

Instructions

- In a medium bowl, cream together the sweetener, butter, and vanilla until well blended.
- Stir in the almond flour, ground hazelnuts, and salt until a firm dough is formed.
- Roll the dough into a 2-inch cylinder and wrap it in plastic wrap. Place the dough in the refrigerator for at least 30 minutes until firm.
- Preheat the oven to 350°F (175°C). Line a baking sheet with parchment paper and lightly grease the paper with butter; set aside.
- Unwrap the chilled cylinder, slice the dough into 18 cookies, and place the cookies on the baking sheet.
- Bake the cookies until firm and lightly browned, about 10 minutes.
- Allow the cookies to cool on the baking

sheet for 5 minutes and then transfer them to a wire rack to cool completely.

- Process less expensive whole nuts in a food processor or blender rather than paying for a pre-ground product. Make sure you don't process the nuts in the appliance too long or you'll end up with nut butter.

Nutritional information:

Net carbs: 6% (2 g)

Fiber: 1 g

Fat: 85% (10 g)

Protein: 9% (3 g)

Kcal: 105

Vanilla-Almond Ice Pops
In childhood, nothing was better than a sweet treat on a hot summer day. This is a more elegant ice pop that can be enjoyed after a leisurely barbecue with friends. It features simple vanilla and coconut flavoring, which can

be enhanced with cut fruit if you want a little more texture to the pop. Use inexpensive ice pop molds; they are easily found for a few dollars in most stores.

Ingredients

1 cup heavy (whipping) cream

2 cups almond milk

1 vanilla bean, halved lengthwise

1 cup shredded unsweetened coconut

Instructions

- Place a medium saucepan over medium heat and add the almond milk, heavy cream, and vanilla bean.
- Bring the liquid to a simmer and reduce the heat to low. Continue to simmer for 5 minutes.
- Remove the saucepan from the heat and let the liquid cool.
- Take the vanilla bean out of the liquid and use a knife to scrape the seeds out of the bean into the liquid.
- Stir in the coconut and divide the liquid between the ice pop molds.
- Freeze until solid, about 4 hours, and

enjoy.

Nutritional information:

Net carbs: 10% (4 g)

Fiber: 2 g

Fat: 81% (15 g)

Protein: 9% (3 g)

Kcal: 166

Raspberry Cheesecake

Cheesecake is a sublime dessert experience: tart, sweet, and infinitely velvety on the tongue. This is a crust-free cheesecake featuring plump, ripe raspberries and a distinct vanilla undertone. You can use any type of berry, sliced peaches or plums, or even a tablespoon of cocoa powder to create gorgeous variations. Your imagination is the limit when you have a perfect cheesecake base to use in your experiments.

Ingredients

1/2 cup cream cheese, at room temperature

2/3 cup coconut oil, melted

6 eggs

3 tablespoons granulated sweetener

3/4 cup raspberries

1 teaspoon alcohol-free pure vanilla extract

1/2 teaspoon baking powder

Instructions

- Preheat the oven to 350°F (175ºC). Line an 8-by-8-inch baking dish with parchment paper and set aside.
- In a large bowl, beat together the coconut oil and cream cheese until smooth.
- Beat in the eggs, scraping down the sides of the bowl at least once.
- Beat in the sweetener, vanilla, and baking powder until smooth.
- Spoon the batter into the baking dish and use a spatula to smooth out the top. Scatter the raspberries on top.
- Bake until the center is firm, about 25 to 30 minutes.
- Allow the cheesecake to cool completely before cutting into 12 squares.
  Any type of berry is delicious in this luscious treat, such as blueberries, strawberries, or blackberries. Whenever

possible for your recipes, use seasonal local fruit for the best flavor and color.

Nutritional information:

Net carbs: 4% (3 g)

Fiber: 1 g

Fat: 85% (18 g)

Protein: 11% (6 g)

Kcal: 176

Chapter 12: The 30-Day Meal Plan

Calendar

Sunday	Monday	Tuesday	Wednesday	Thursday	Friday	Saturday
				1	2	3
4	5	6	7	8	9	10
11	12	13	14	15	16	17
18	19	20	21	22	23	24
25	26	27	28	29	30	31

Chapter 12: The 30-Day Meal Plan

12.1

The meal plan is meant to serve as a guide, so it's not compulsory you follow this, you can adjust it to fit your taste and schedule using the recipes earlier that were discussed in the previous chapters.

Some of the recipes are easy and straightforward to prepare while some others require early and proper planning, so put that into consideration as you start the diet.

12.2

Having a meal plan at the start of your diet gives you higher chances of success. A meal plan gives you a sense of direction. Many times, people give up because they don't have a good plan in place.

A meal plan in place means you have an idea of

what you're eating as your next meal. This is key to achieving success as many people give up because they usually don't have a good meal plan in place.

The meal plan is what sustains you on the keto diet. Many out there are complaining about how they tried the diet for some time and because they weren't seeing any changes

DAY 1

Breakfast: Avocado and Eggs

Snack: Spinach-Blueberry Smoothie

Lunch: Cauliflower Cheddar Soup (leftovers)

Snack: Nutty Shortbread Cookies

Dinner: Baked Coconut Haddock and Brussels Sprouts Casserole

DAY 2

Breakfast: Lemon-Cashew Smoothie

Snack: Almond Butter Fudge

Lunch: BLT Salad

Snack: Bacon-Pepper Fat Bombs

Dinner: Roasted Pork Loin with Grainy Mustard Sauce and Golden Rosti

DAY 3

Breakfast: Peanut Butter Cup Smoothie

Snack: Walnut Herb-Crusted Goat Cheese

Lunch: Cauliflower-Cheddar Soup

Snack: Bacon-Cheese Deviled Eggs

Dinner: Lamb Leg with Sun-Dried Tomato Pesto (leftovers) and Sautéed Crispy Zucchini

DAY 4

Breakfast: Nut Medley Granola

Snack: Bacon-Cheese Deviled Eggs

Lunch: Chicken-Avocado Lettuce Wraps

Snack: Creamy Cinnamon Smoothie

Dinner: Lamb Leg with Sun-Dried Tomato Pesto and Cheesy Mashed Cauliflower

DAY 5

Breakfast: Nut Medley Granola

Snack: Smoked Salmon Fat Bombs

Lunch: Breakfast Bake

Snack: Almond Butter Fudge

Dinner: Chicken Bacon Burger and Portobello Mushroom Pizza

DAY 6

Breakfast: Berry Green Smoothie

Snack: Bacon-Pepper Fat Bombs

Lunch: Roasted Pork Loin with Grainy Mustard Sauce (leftovers)

Snack: Vanilla-Almond Ice Pops

Dinner: Turkey Meatloaf and Golden Rosti

DAY 7

Breakfast: Breakfast Bake

Snack: Creamy Cinnamon Smoothie

Lunch: Turkey Meatloaf (leftovers)

Snack: Nutty Shortbread Cookies

Dinner: Cheesy Garlic Salmon and Garlicky Green Beans

DAY 8

Breakfast: Peanut Butter Cup Smoothie

Snack: Crispy Parmesan Crackers

Lunch: BLT Salad

Snack: Smoked Salmon Fat Bombs

Dinner: Lamb Leg with Sun-Dried Tomato Pesto (leftovers) and Cheesy Mashed Cauliflower

DAY 9

Breakfast: Avocado and Eggs

Snack: Almond Butter Fudge

Lunch: Cauliflower-Cheddar Soup

Snack: Berry Green Smoothie

Dinner: Herb Butter Scallops and Pesto Zucchini Noodles

DAY 10

Breakfast: Nut Medley Granola

Snack: Vanilla-Almond Ice Pops

Lunch: Crab Salad-Stuffed Avocado

Snack: Chocolate-Coconut Treats

Dinner: Lamb Leg with Sun-Dried Tomato Pesto and Brussels Sprouts Casserole

DAY 11

Breakfast: Berry Green Smoothie

Snack: Nutty Shortbread Cookies

Lunch: Chicken-Avocado Lettuce Wraps

Snack: Crispy Parmesan Crackers

Dinner: Baked Coconut Haddock and Brussels Sprouts Casserole

DAY 12

Breakfast: Breakfast Bake

Snack: Queso Dip

Lunch: Roasted Pork Loin with Grainy Mustard Sauce (leftovers)

Snack: Almond Butter Fudge

Dinner: Lemon Butter Chicken and Sautéed Asparagus with Walnuts

DAY 13

Breakfast: Nut Medley Granola

Snack: Chicken-Avocado Lettuce Wraps

Lunch: Breakfast Bake

Snack: Raspberry Cheesecake with 1/4 cup whipped cream

Dinner: Turkey Meatloaf and Creamed Spinach

DAY 14

Breakfast: Lemon-Cashew Smoothie

Snack: Peanut Butter Mousse

Lunch: Cauliflower-Cheddar Soup (leftovers)

Snack: Chocolate-Coconut Treats

Dinner: Roasted Pork Loin with Grainy Mustard Sauce and Mushrooms with Camembert

DAY 15

Breakfast: Breakfast Bake

Snack: Almond Butter Fudge

Lunch: Chicken-Avocado Lettuce Wraps

Snack: Nutty Shortbread Cookies

Dinner: Lemon Butter Chicken and Sautéed Asparagus with Walnuts

DAY 16

Breakfast: Avocado and Eggs

Snack: Bacon-Pepper Fat Bombs

Lunch: Lemon-Cashew Smoothie

Snack: Almond Butter Fudge

Dinner: Baked Coconut Haddock and Brussels Sprouts Casserole

DAY 17

Breakfast: Avocado and Eggs

Snack: Crispy Parmesan Crackers

Lunch: Chicken-Avocado Lettuce Wraps

Snack: Queso Dip

Dinner: Turkey Meatloaf and Creamed Spinach

DAY 18

Breakfast: Berry Green Smoothie

Snack: Raspberry Cheesecake with 1/4 cup whipped cream

Lunch: BLT Salad

Snack: Crispy Parmesan Crackers

Dinner: Roasted Pork Loin with Grainy Mustard Sauce and Mushrooms with Camembert

DAY 19

Breakfast: Creamy Cinnamon Smoothie

Snack: Chocolate-Coconut Treats

Lunch: Cauliflower-Cheddar Soup

Snack: Vanilla-Almond Ice Pops

Dinner: Herb Butter Scallops and Pesto Zucchini Noodles

DAY 20

Breakfast: Peanut Butter Cup Smoothie

Snack: Almond Butter Fudge

Lunch: Crab Salad-Stuffed Avocado

Snack: Nutty Shortbread Cookies

Dinner: Baked Coconut Haddock and Brussels Sprouts Casserole

DAY 21

Breakfast: Lemon-Cashew Smoothie

Snack: Berry Green Smoothie

Lunch: Roasted Pork Loin with Grainy Mustard Sauce (leftovers)

Snack: BLT Salad

Dinner: Turkey Meatloaf and Creamed Spinach

DAY 22

Breakfast: Avocado and Eggs

Snack: Bacon-Pepper Fat Bombs

Lunch: Turkey Meatloaf (leftovers)

Snack: Walnut Herb-Crusted Goat Cheese

Dinner: Roasted Pork Loin with Grainy Mustard Sauce and Golden Rosti

DAY 23

Breakfast: Creamy Cinnamon Smoothie

Snack: Nutty Shortbread Cookies

Lunch: Crab Salad-Stuffed Avocado

Snack: Berry Green Smoothie

Dinner: Roasted Pork Loin with Grainy Mustard Sauce and Mushrooms with Camembert

DAY 24

Breakfast: Breakfast Bake

Snack: Berry Green Smoothie

Lunch: Chocolate-Coconut Treats

Snack: BLT Salad

Dinner: Herb Butter Scallops and Pesto Zucchini Noodles

DAY 25

Breakfast: Peanut Butter Cup Smoothie

Snack: Nutty Shortbread Cookies

Lunch: Creamy Cinnamon Smoothie

Snack: Vanilla-Almond Ice Pops

Dinner: Turkey Meatloaf and Creamed Spinach

DAY 26

Breakfast: Berry Green Smoothie

Snack: BLT Salad

Lunch: Cauliflower-Cheddar Soup

Snack: Raspberry Cheesecake with 1/4 cup whipped cream

Dinner: Lamb Leg with Sun-Dried Tomato Pesto (leftovers) and Cheesy Mashed

Cauliflower

DAY 27

Breakfast: Creamy Cinnamon Smoothie

Snack: Crispy Parmesan Crackers

Lunch: Crab Salad-Stuffed Avocado

Snack: Queso Dip

Dinner: Lemon Butter Chicken and Sautéed Asparagus with Walnuts

DAY 28

Breakfast: Crispy Parmesan Crackers

Snack: Nutty Shortbread Cookies

Lunch: Chicken-Avocado Lettuce Wraps

Snack: Almond Butter Fudge

Dinner: Lemon Butter Chicken and Sautéed Asparagus with Walnuts

DAY 29

Breakfast: Creamy Cinnamon Smoothie

Snack: Chocolate-Coconut Treats

Lunch: Cauliflower-Cheddar Soup

Snack: Vanilla-Almond Ice Pops

Dinner: Herb Butter Scallops and Pesto Zucchini Noodles

DAY 30

Breakfast: Lemon-Cashew Smoothie

Snack: Peanut Butter Mousse

Lunch: Cauliflower-Cheddar Soup (leftovers)

Snack: Chocolate-Coconut Treats

Dinner: Roasted Pork Loin with Grainy Mustard Sauce and Mushrooms with Camembert

12.3

How to use the meal plan:

- You should start thinking and planning for your meals at least 3 days before. Don't just choose recipes in an undeliberate manner, it is smart to actually choose recipes you're a bit familiar alongside the new ones. This way you won't feel overwhelmed.
- Using the guideline, you should have a daily consumption of about 1500 to 1900 calories. If you don't have an idea how many calories you are meant to eat, check using an online macro calculator. In a case where you need more calories than what is available in the meal plan, you can switch any of the meals for one with

higher calories or you can also add more oil or an ingredient while cooking.
- This meal plan is designed for one person. This means that if you want to use them for more people, all you need to do is multiply the quantity of ingredients by the number of people.
- Since some of the recipes in the meal plan might not be meals you used to cook prior to this time, you should shop for your ingredients earlier than when you need them. You could start shopping over the weekend. You don't have to take a very big list to the store for shopping, simply start by planning for the first week.
- Prepare the ingredients that need to prepped beforehand.
- If you're on a very strict keto diet, ensure you tweak this meal plan to make it work for you.
- If you are allergic to any ingredient, ensure you replace them with other low-carb substitutes.

Your Quick-Start Action Step:

Draft your meal plan and find out how much it will cost you to prepare the recipes in your meal plan. This is an important part of becoming successful with the diet.

Chapter 13: How to Dine Out with the Keto Diet

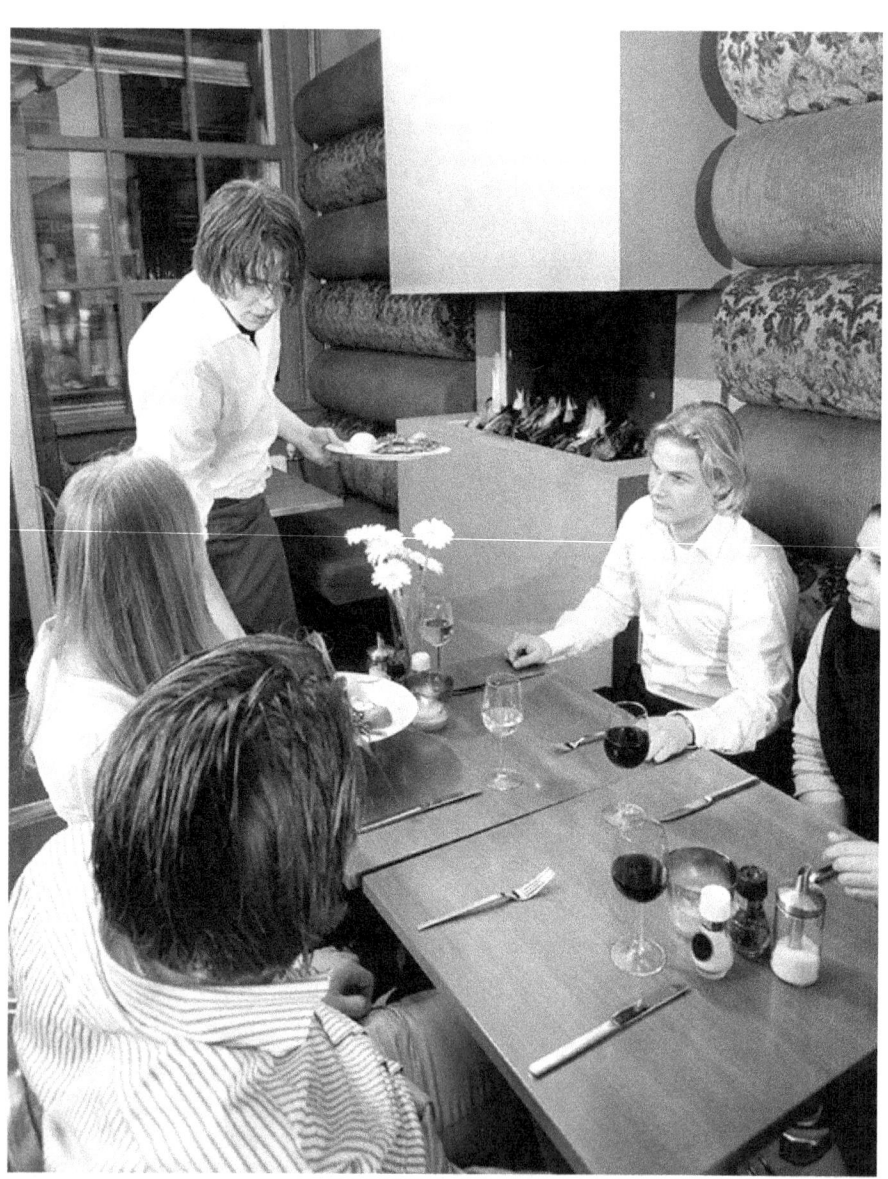

Chapter 13: How to Dine Out with the Keto Diet

This is a guide to ensure that even though you are having dinner anywhere, you still maintain your keto diet. It is very possible to obtain low-carb food anywhere. Below are some tips to help with enjoying a delicious meal anywhere and yet not compromising your diet lifestyle:

- Make a sacred oath – this is arguably the most important tip to ensure you don't compromise your diet lifestyle while dining out. Before putting yourself in such a situation, make a commitment to strictly avoid the big offenders (carbs).
- Ditch the starch – avoid the bread, the pasta, the potatoes, and the rice. It's better to keep all temptation off your plate by not even ordering the starchy food in the first place. If after such careful ordering your order still arrives with a starchy side, then weigh your options. If you are confident and sure that you will leave it untouched, then you can go on

with feasting, but if you feel the craving to "just taste some," then you should request for your meal to be replaced with something that contains no starch, and if you don't want to draw unnecessary attention to yourself then you can find a way to discard the unwanted pieces of your food in the nearest bin.

- Embrace healthy fat –take fate into your hands whenever you visit a restaurant; you can request extra butter and let it melt on your meat or veggie. When your meal contains salad, you can request olive oil and vinegar dressing.
- Pay more attention to protein, vegetables and fats; it is important to focus on the healthy food, as long as your mind is fixated on them, your cravings for the other unsafe foods will be reduced. It is relatively easy to obtain healthy fats to add to your plates. Example of these include butter, olive oil, and sour cream. You can request them if you don't see them.

- Be very careful when choosing your drink; some drinks are perfectly fine and completely safe, for example; tea, coffee, or water. Some alcoholic beverages are also fine, like dry wine, light beer, or champagne.
- Watch out for condiments and sauces; some sauces have a very high fat content, for example, like Béarnaise sauce, while others consist mostly of carbs, like ketchup. If you are not certain of the content of the sauce you're given, then ask, and avoid it if it consists mostly of sugar or flour.
- Is dessert really necessary – you don't need to order dessert unless it's really required; you can just stick with a cup of coffee while others can finish their sweets. If you feel your coffee is hardly satisfying then adding butter or cream to it is enough to satiate your need.
- Be patient – get into the dinner conversation, remember to stay hydrated, and enjoy your tea or coffee.

Usually, being on a keto diet means that it may eat a bit of a while before you are satisfied; however, don't give in to the need to eat in overdrive—this won't help if you're trying to lose weight. Give it some time; you might eventually feel satisfied.

- Ensure you ease the edge your hunger before leaving home; it is only safe to eat a fatty snack before leaving for the party. You can pick olives, nuts or cheese, any of these are good choices. This makes it much easier to say no to the big offenders (starchy foods).

Chapter 14: Mistakes to Avoid When on the Keto Diet

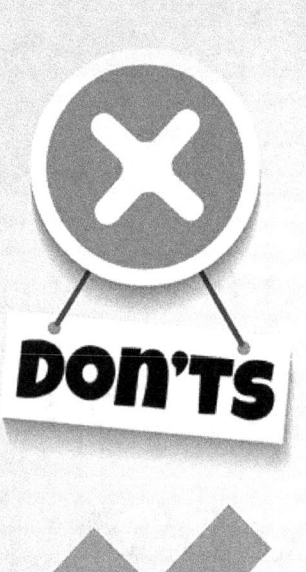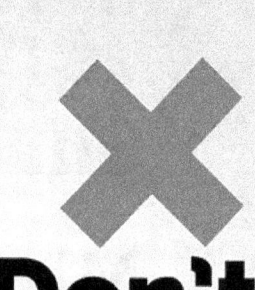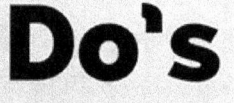

Chapter 14: Mistakes To Avoid When On A Keto Diet

Being on a ketogenic diet is not so easy. It requires a whole lot of commitment and focus since it entails you changing your normal routine. Your body is going to undergo an internal change, and your normal daily activities will have to change too. Many people, upon being on a keto diet, do not see results as fast as they hope, while others really love it. What makes the difference is certain common mistakes that people make when beginning a ketogenic diet. This is fine, as no one is really perfect and mistakes do happen. We must all learn that mistakes are to be learned from in other to avoid making them again.

Below are some of the common mistakes that people make when staying on a keto diet. This will help you avoid these mistakes as you continue on your keto diet journey.

- Doing keto as a quick fix – the keto diet is not a quick fix to solve your body issues. It is a new way of life that you have to stick to and be consistent with in order to see results. You may notice some fast changes as soon as you start a keto diet but this doesn't mean you can go right back to your old eating habits and still expect these changes to remain. It's very likely you'll go back to how you were before, with all those changes completely lost. Do not expect that such changes are going to be permanent just by being loyal to keto for a couple of months.
- Worrying too much over the scale – it is true that one of the benefits of being on a keto diet is that it helps with weight loss, helping burn stored-up body fat. However, it is important to note that this is a process that takes time and being too fixated and obsessed over your weight is going to

make it look longer and harder. Frequently checking your weight is not going to help, whether multiple times a day or even daily. You just have to trust that since you are doing things the right way, then results are bound to come, and that staying off carbs and hitting your macros daily is going to make your weight come off. Constant checking of your weight only puts a heavy weight on your mind and leaves you discouraged. Significant changes occur over multiple weeks or months. It is advisable to only check your weight once a week.

- Fear of fats – it sounds like an oxymoron to say that you actually have to eat fat to lose fat, but this is true and actually works. When staying on a keto diet, it is quite important to eat a large amount of fat to ensure your body reaches the set goal. Fat is not bad for you when on a keto diet, and when you calculate your macros and discover the large amount of fat you have to consume, don't be afraid. Fat must contribute up to 75 percent of your diet when on a ketogenic diet; this is how you can be successful with it. So understanding that this amount of fat is going to help, will make you not afraid but rather help you in embracing high fat consumption.

- Consuming the wrong type of fat – eating fat when on a keto diet is very essential, but you must ensure that you're eating the right type of fat. There are good fats to embrace and bad fats to avoid when starting a keto diet; don't just assume that since you require a large fat content in your diet then all fats are good for you. The bad fats are the processed fats—they are present in processed vegetable oils. Therefore, cooking with these oils is a big fat no. The good fats that you need are the monounsaturated fats, naturally occurring trans-fats, saturated fats, and the polyunsaturated fats. Getting these types of fats is easy. The good fats are present in foods like avocados, walnuts, eggs, butter, etc. When these are added to your diet, you'll realize than not only are you meeting the fat requirements of your body but you're also sticking with the good fats.

- Consuming excess protein in your diet – some do not see this as a problem when staying on a keto diet; they see this as a substitute for their low-carb diet. However, it is important to note that having too much protein in your diet will have certain undesirable effects on your body. When an excess amount of protein is consumed, the body only utilizes the amount it requires while the remaining is converted to fat, storing it up in the body; this is bad as reducing weight is what we want to achieve and not the exact opposite. It is very simple to avoid this: all you need do is simply to focus more on your macros so as not to have an excessive intake of anything.

- Not drinking enough water – when doing the keto diet, one of the internal changes that your body undergoes is loss of body fluids. To counter this, it is very important to stay hydrated by drinking a lot of water. When you're not staying hydrated, your body is going to respond by storing a lot of fat; again, this is bad as reducing weight is what we want to achieve and not the exact opposite. When you lose body fluids and electrolytes when on a keto diet, it can easily be replenished by consuming a large quantity of water. This will also help your body organs function properly and your body work effectively. Some individuals aren't comfortable with drinking a lot of water daily but this is something that has to be strictly followed if you want to see the changes that you desire. Usually, one gallon of water per day is recommended.

- Not having enough sleep – when your body begins to enter a state of ketosis and fat becomes your body's primary source of energy (as is usually the case when one is on a keto diet), it is normal that your body doesn't get as much sleep as before when you were still following your old eating habits. You therefore need to try, as much as possible, to get the right amount of sleep that you require. You need sleep, and getting the right amount is important, as not getting the right amount will affect the overall functioning of your body. When you get the right amount of sleep, it enables your body to cope with the numerous changes it undergoes as a result of being on a keto diet.

- Eating the same thing all the time – when on a keto diet, since you're restricted in the amounts of carb you can consume, it may give you the idea that you are also restricted in the number of recipes you can have as well. Because of this, some people seem to eat a monotonous meal, eating the same things all the time. When you mix things up properly, you will discover that your meal can actually be quite enjoyable. This will help in being consistent with staying on a ketogenic diet and not being discouraged; it allows you to want to go further with the diet as it keeps your morale high. It is okay to add in some low-carb vegetables to your diet every once in a while. You should ensure to keep your taste buds excited so even your favorite meal doesn't begin to taste bland due to eating it too often and you begin to get sick of it.

- Using others as a yardstick for yourself – this is a mental mistake but with a large effect on whether you are consistent with the keto diet or give up too quickly. It is a part of human nature to compare yourself with others; people love doing it and everyone does it. When on a ketogenic diet, you can't afford to compare yourself with others; your focus should be on your body and no one else as otherwise it will be like signing your own death warrant. The response of everyone's body to the diet differs with individuals; this means that people are going to experience changes in their body at different times and at different rates from yours. So simply focus more on your own body changes and trust that, since you're doing the right thing, your weight loss will come and you will reach your goal.

Most of these mistakes are easily avoided; some of them are physical while some are mostly mental. The mental ones are the hardest to avoid. Once you notice that you have made any of these mistakes just ensure that you take a step back, evaluate the situation, find out where the mistake came from, determine how it can be solved, and get right back to things.

Bonus Chapter: Other Types of the Keto Diet

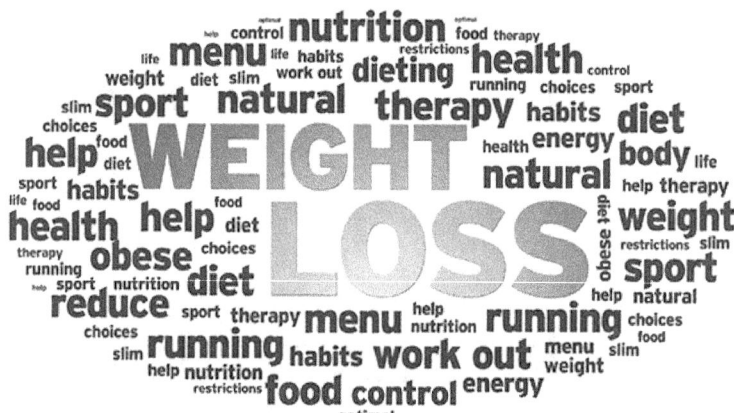

Bonus Chapter: Other Types of the Keto Diet

15.1

The focus of this book is on the standard keto diet, however, there are other types of diets out there. Your goal and activity level will determine what type of ketogenic diet is best for you. You may have to try the different types out to find out which works well for you. There are other types namely; the Targeted, Cyclical and the High Protein ketogenic diet.

The Targeted Ketogenic Diet is best for keeping up with exercise performance, energizing your muscles with a good amount of glucose during exercise. For someone who wants to try the targeted ketogenic diet, you should consume about 25 to 50 grams of net carbs up to 30 minutes or an hour before exercise, and then follow the standard ketogenic diet every other time. The targeted variant is best for two categories of people; people who require carbs for energy during exercise but cannot afford to have long loads of carb that the cyclical ketogenic diet offers, individuals who are just starting an exercise program and cannot afford to do the required amount of exercise to fully optimize a cyclical diet. However, people who have not tried the standard diet for at least one or two months are advised to not try this diet.

The Cyclical Ketogenic Diet combines the standard keto diet with carb loading days. It is usually used by people who have more intense exercise activities for example athletes and bodybuilders, this is because to optimize their performance during training, high volume and intensity is required. This diet makes it almost possible for them to be at their best while engaging in such voluminous and intense exercise. However, it is not recommended for people who are not well adapted to keto yet.

The High Protein Ketogenic Diet requires increasing the intake of protein. It's best for older people who stand high risks of muscle breakdown or people who need more protein to protect muscle mass like bodybuilders. It is equally a great choice for people who show signs of being deficient in protein. Such signs include thinning hair or loss or muscle. Individuals with kidney diseases and those who want to get on the keto diet for therapeutic reasons should not go on the high protein diet.

15.2 Each of the other types of the ketogenic diet comes with their benefits and are discussed shortly below.

Benefits of the Targeted Ketogenic Diet

While on the targeted keto diet, you can perform highly intense activities and yet not have to be out of ketosis for long periods of time. In other words, it increases energy levels for athletes and people who do strenuous exercises.

Going on the targeted keto diet can also be helpful to athletes in that it boosts the insulin level which prevents muscle break down and rather promotes muscle growth.

Benefits of the High Protein Ketogenic Diet

The high protein keto diet is helpful for achieving greater results with weight loss, this is also linked with the fact that it reduces hunger level. It has equally been proven to helpful in managing diabetes because it improves glycemic control in patients who have type-2 diabetes.

Benefits of the Cyclical Ketogenic Diet

The cyclical keto diet uses anabolic "growth" hormones like insulin to help athletes gain muscle as well as replenish the glycogen available in the body to enable them lift heavier weights.

The cyclical keto diet has also been proven to be helpful in restoring adrenals and revitalizing the thyroid.

15.3 Take some time and do a study on each of the types of the keto diet mentioned here. There's quite a volume of information available online about them, go online and read up.

Ketogenic Diet Conversion Tables

Liquid Volumes		
Ml	U.S.	Fl oz.
15	1 tbsp	½
30	1/8 c	1
60	1/4 c	2
118	1/2 c	4
177	3/4 c	6
237	1 c	8
355	1 1/2 c	12
474	2 c	16
710	3 c	24
746	4 c	32

Dry weights

Grams	Oz – lb
28	1
57	2
85	3
113	4 oz – 1/4 lb
151	1/3 lb
227	8 oz – 1/2 lb
302	2/3 lb
340	12 oz – 3/4 lb
454	1 lb
907	2 lb

OVEN TEMPERATURES	
Celsius	Fahrenheit
140°	285°
150°	300°

160°	320°
170°	338°
180°	356°
200°	392°
220°	425°
225°	437°

Bonus Book Preview: "Keto Meal Prep for Beginners: Your Essential Ketogenic Diet Easy Meal Plan to Save Time & Money for Long-Term Weight Loss, Eating Better and Healthy Living" by Amy Maria Adams

Chapter 3: Easy Steps to Meal Prepping

Keto Meal Prep Planning Steps

1. *Plan the Meal Prep*

Planning entails picking a day for keto meal prepping, picking the meals you want for the week, and settling on the right recipes for the meals.

- *Pick the prepping day.*

    The first thing to do is to pick the day for prepping the meals. Sunday is the best day because most people are off work and can enlist the help of others if you want. Some people opt for two days in a week to prep, which allows them to split meal prepping into two, usually Sunday and Wednesday.

- *Choose the meals.*

    Once you have a day or have decided to split meal prepping into two days, choose the meals you want. Since we are focused on planning for a whole week, choose all the meals, desserts, and snack that you want.

Ensure that the meals are healthy and are keto compliant. You can also mark the meals on a calendar at this point.

- *Pick meal recipes.*

Once you know the meals you want, the next thing to do is to find keto recipes for the meals you have chosen. Keep the calories and macros in mind when picking the recipes so that you balance the meals correctly.

Beginners should choose easy recipes with a few ingredients. Even better, go for recipes that have similar ingredients—for instance, different meals with meats or vegetables—to make shopping and cooking easier.

Knowledge of how macronutrients are converted into calories will help you keep the right ratios. When choosing recipes, select the ones that you want to eat and will enjoy.

It should not just be healthy, you should be happy about it.

- *Write down the week's keto menu.*

Once you have the recipes, write them down in the order you want to eat them during the week. Write down or print out the recipes so that you have them to follow on prep day. It also helps to craft the order in which the food is prepared. Start with the more engaging meals and finish up with the easy ones, like those for breakfast, desserts, and snacks.

- *Pick a prep day.*

This is the point where you decide if you want to do it on Saturday or Sunday or if you want to prep twice, say on Wednesday and Sunday. As advised earlier, it works best to prep a day after shopping, or you can choose to prep the same day you shop.

2. *Write Down the Shopping List*

Draw a shopping list of the ingredients from each of the recipes you have settled on. Break down the list into food categories—dairy, meat, vegetables, etc. The list must have the exact quantities of each ingredient as per the keto recipes. Avoid packaged and processed products.

Tip: Always check your fridge, freezer, and pantry to confirm what you have so that you do not overstock.

3. Go Shopping for the Items You Listed

Once you have the shopping list, all you have left is to buy what you need before you embark on the actual prepping. As said earlier, pick a convenient shopping day and time so that you are not drained by the experience. Shop when there is less traffic in the shops so that you will easily get what you want to leave.

Apart from the recipe items, buy the keto pantry essentials we listed earlier—any kitchen equipment and storage containers enough for the meals you will be preparing. Make sure you have your shopping list and stick to buying the items in it as planned.

4. Cook and Store the Meals

This is the point you have been preparing for—making the effort count and turning the recipes into delicious meals. Have all ingredients ready and the recipes out when doing this and follow them step by step.

Cooking can be tricky and may take longer than planned or suggested by the respective recipes, but keep going. It will be easier as you go along. Read through the recipes to understand what you need to do and how to do it. It is a good idea to start with those meals with the longest preparation process.

Those that need to be marinated or simmered for long periods should be dealt with first before the cooking day or hour so that everything is ready for the finalization of the dishes. All the veggies and meats that need to be prepared (cutting, slicing, dicing, marinating, etc.) should be done earlier so that they are ready on your cooking day. You may want to do this on shopping day after making your purchases or very early in the morning on prep day.

When packing the foods for storage, take into account the storage life of the various constituents of the meals packed, as well as recommended refrigeration times after cooking. For example, cut vegetables, like onions and peppers, will stay fresh under refrigeration for up to three days. Leafy vegetable if dried will last about a week, and cooked grains and meat dishes should be eaten within four days of cooking. Warm the meals at respective healthy temperatures when eating.

Tips:

- o Newbies to keto and to meal prep should begin small and gradually prepare more meals once they learn and identify their favorite recipes and get a handle on meal prepping respectively.

- When you start, choose simple recipes with a few ingredients and pick recipes with similar ingredients to shorten your shopping list and make cooking faster.

- If you are a beginner, you do not have to do a whole week. Try preparing three meals for starters to have a feel of the process.

- Start with some recipes that you have prepared before.

- Plan meals around seasonal produce for freshness and price value.

- Preparing the same dish for two or three mealtimes is a good energy-saving and time-saving idea for beginners.

Quick Start Action Step

Meal prepping is not a complicated process, is it? It may seem like at first, especially for a beginner when you move from reading to actual doing.

Now what you need to do is to act on the steps learned here and follow through on the keto meal prep planning. Pick the meals you want and decide the meal prep day. Draw your shopping list to cover the ingredients, buy everything you need, and finally cook your meals and store them for the week ahead. There is no better satisfaction than eating a delicious healthy meal prepared by yourself.

Chapter 6: Keto Meal Prep on a Budget

As much as there is a perception out there that the ketogenic diet is expensive, it isn't really true. It is possible to be on a keto diet comfortably on a budget. We shall learn in this chapter how to do keto meal prep on a budget of $50 weekly or even less.

The truth is, there are expensive ingredients for some recipes that can make it an expensive affair. The classic low-carb keto foods, like meat, leafy vegetables, and high-fat fish can be expensive. However, for every one of the expensive ingredients, there are high-quality alternatives and substitutes that you can cook with that keep in mind the nutritional requirements of keto.

Keto on a diet simply needs a bit of ingenuity and planning to get it done. By the end of this chapter, you will know how to eat a high-quality ketogenic diet on a budget. With some of the money-saving tips already discussed and the insights you will get here, you should hack the keto diet on a budget.

There are so many tricks available to you, like buying supplies in bulk, looking for deals and discounts, and shopping at farm markets, which guarantee you savings and will easily support you if you are on a budget.

The benefits of keto diet on a budget:

- You will be able to stay on the diet despite low finances.
- There are still high-quality recipe alternatives and substitutes.
- Saves you money.
- You will still get the required calories and macros.
- You do not have to strain financially.
- No stress from lack of money to by the high-priced recipe items.

6.1 How to Succeed on a $50-a-Week Keto Meal Prep Plan

Here are some great ideas to help you to achieve a keto meal prep on $50 for a week of keto meals:

- **Plan in advance.**

Apart from keeping your meal plan simple, this is the most important point for cost-saving.

Planning will save you money through the whole process—from purchase to restocking.

Planning prevents impulse and unnecessary purchases because you will have to shop as per a predetermined list.

- **Opt for cheaper ingredient alternatives or substitutes.**

Always go for cheaper recipe alternatives to the more expensive seasonal or classic recipe ingredients. There are high-priced and low-priced items for each food or ingredient category.

- *Cheese*

    This is a staple of the keto diet. Avoid specialty cheeses and buy a block of regular cheese and grate or shred it yourself.

- *Fish*

    Fish is a high-quality and healthy keto fat and protein source but is often expensive.

Use canned fish in place of fresh fish if you are on a diet.

- *Poultry*

    If you have to buy chicken in parts, go for the cheaper cuts like thighs, legs, and wings. Alternatively, buy a whole chicken which is cheaper than buying parts.

- *Meat*

    Go for fatty meat cuts. They are cheaper than lean cuts, and buy from a butchery rather than a supermarket.

- *Vegetables*

    Vegetables are integral to the success of the keto diet. Buy frozen vegetables instead of fresh low-carb vegetables, which are usually expensive at supermarkets. Frozen vegetables are cheap and do not go bad as fast as fresh vegetables.

- *Eggs*

Stock a lot of eggs in your pantry. They are one of the cheaper protein sources and are versatile for keto recipes.

- **Shop in bulk.**

There is no better way of saving money or working within a budget that shopping for ingredients in bulk because it is cheaper. Stock up items on sale every time you come across them.

- **Be on the lookout for price discounts and offer.**

If you are on a budget, be on the lookout for price reductions and deals on quantities. This is a great way of getting more for less.

- **Avoid impulse buying.**

Simply put, do not purchase anything that you do not have on your shopping list; otherwise, you will mess up your budget.

- **Buy items online.**

Items are generally cheaper online. Take advantage of online stores to save money and get more items for at your weekly budget. You will be amazed at how much you save and get by buying things online than at the local supermarket.

- **Keep your meal prep simple.**

The simpler your keto meal plan is, the cheaper and easier it will be on your finances.

Tip: Do not buy a product or ingredient you have never used before in bulk because it may not be what you like or want. Buy a little to try and only buy in bulk if it is something for you.

Quick Start Action Step

Sticking to a keto diet on a $50-per-week meal plan is possible. You can even spend less depending on your preferences and meals choices. Use the insights in this chapter and take the simple options above to keep you healthy on keto when you are on a budget.

Chapter 7: Keto Meal Prep for Weight Loss

As you are now aware, the ketogenic diet can be used for putting on weight, for maintaining the weight you are at, or for losing weight. For each of the three options, there are different and specific keto calories and macros that are effective and recommended for desired results.

Fat burning for weight loss is one of the main benefits of ketosis and is probably the reason why it is so popular. Keto makes people feel great and more satiated, which helps you to eat less of what you should not eat. It elevates mental and physical energy, which should not be impeded by low finances.

Achieving weight loss through keto on a lean budget is possible, and you should still be able to buy the weight-loss ingredients within your budget. Much of it is similar to what we have discussed in the previous chapter but directed at keto items for weight loss.

There are many keto weight-loss recipes and ingredients that can be cooked and bought respectively without spending so much money. Since dieting is about nutrition content in an ingredient of food, you will find nutrient-rich foods that are not necessarily in the high-price bracket. Make your pick from the list of affordable keto weight-loss ingredients further down.

7.1 Benefits of Keto Meal Pep for Weight Loss

The following are the foremost benefits of keto meal planning for weight loss:

- It elevates mental focus and concentration.
- It is highly effective at burning fat.
- It infuses your body and muscles with energy.
- It curtails constant hunger pangs.
- It helps in blood sugar balance and regulation.
- It improves skin health and fights acne.
- It controls cholesterol and triglyceride levels.
- It improves hormonal regulation in women, especially for severe PMS symptoms.

7.2 Affordable Weight-Loss Ingredients for Keto Meal Prep on a Budget

The following are great affordable keto weight-loss ingredients for one on a budget:

1. *Avocado*

Avocado is a ketogenic diet essential for healthy fat content, minerals, and vitamins. Not only is it good for its rich fat content but it also helps keto beginners to deal with symptoms of keto flu. It is high in fat and very low on carbs.

2. *Kimchi and sauerkraut*

Fermented foods carrying good bacteria, and prebiotic fibers are good for gut health. Studies have found that a healthy bacteria balance in your stomach can help to reduce fat mass.

3. *Eggs*

Eggs are the most versatile keto foods and one of the healthiest proteins for weight loss. Eggs will leave you feeling full and will keep you from packing extra calories.

4. *Garlic*

Garlic, as you know, has many long-exploited health benefits. A study found that garlic can help with weight loss.

5. *Leafy vegetables*

Collard greens, kale, spinach, and Swiss chard are great and affordable keto weight-loss foods. They are high in fiber, which slows digestion and iron nutrients which helps the body absorb the nutrients efficiently.

6. *Nuts*

Nuts are high in healthy fat and are not fattening as you may think. Look for recipes that incorporate them. Nuts improve metabolism and help with weight loss because of the high fiber content, which leaves you with a feeling of being full, thus keeping you from eating. Here are the best nuts:

- Almonds (carbs: 6 grams)
- Brazil nuts (carbs: 3 grams)

- Cashews (carbs: 9 grams)
- Macadamia nuts (carbs: 4 grams)
- Pecans (carbs: 4 grams)
- Pistachios (carbs: 8 grams)
- Walnuts (carbs: 4 grams)

7. *Protein powder*

Use protein powder to complement and supplement protein in your meals. Get protein benefits without extra calories—no extra fat or carbohydrates.

8. *Vinegar*

Use vinegar to replace high-calorie additions or condiments to your food.

9. *Pasture-raised chicken*

Eat free-range chicken and benefit from the fat-loss benefits of protein.

10. *Cruciferous vegetables*

Vegetables such as broccoli and cauliflower fall in this group and are keto staples because of their weight-loss benefits. They are a source of sulforaphane and fiber. Sulforaphane has been linked with stimulating energy-burning brown fat and improving gut health. It is also linked to fighting obesity.

11. *Olives and olive oil*

Olive oil helps with fat loss and promotes a leaner body. The healthy fats in olive oil and its anti-inflammatory properties are key to weight loss.

12. *Chilies*

Chilies have fat-burning properties, which are why obesity is low among people who consume a lot of chilies. Chilies contain capsaicin, which reduces appetite and boosts the burning of body fat.

13. *Coconut oil*

Coconut oil has healthy fats and promotes fat loss. A study of obese men found that supplementing their diet with two tablespoons (30 mL) of coconut oil daily helped them cut their waistlines by one inch.

These are some of the top keto ingredients that you can get easily when you are working with a tight grocery budget to help you with keto meal prep for weight loss.

Quick Start Action Step

Pick some of these keto ingredients to help you make the most out of your keto meal prep for weight loss.

Chapter 8: Keto Meal Prep—Mistakes to Avoid

There are some common mistakes that people make on the keto diet that should be avoided because you will never succeed if you keep them up. In fact, it is possible to make some of these mistakes without knowing it. Keto meal prep is really effective if you stick to the script.

Keto does not have to drain your wallet. Doing things the correct way will help you see great returns on investment. Planning and preparation are key to making keto meal prepping very easy, and it ensures success.

8.1 Common Keto Mistakes

The following are some of the common keto meal prep mistakes you want to avoid:

1. Lack of Proper Planning

We already discussed the importance of planning for keto meal prepping. Lack of planning means that you open the doors for many things to go wrong. Failing to prepare means you should prepare to fail.

If you do not plan, you will eat the wrong things, waste time, and lose value for your money. An essential part of planning is doing extensive research into the ingredients and recipes you want to cook.

2. Eating Too Much Protein

You know the macro ratios required for successful ketosis. Eating too much protein is very easy and is a common mistake that must be suppressed. Too much protein consumption leads to elevated blood sugar because it is converted into glucose and defeating ketosis.

3. Low Mineral Intake

Ketosis increases acid production in the body, which lowers the body pH. Basic food minerals help balance out this state and create a normal pH.

4. Not Eating Enough Fat

Keto relies on fat for body energy; if you do not eat enough, you are putting a strain on the body, especially because you have cut on the other energy sources of the body.

5. Tracking on Carbohydrate Intake

Many people quickly forget that they should be tracking everything they eat and only track carb macros in the endeavor to reduce the carbs they consume. When you track only one macro, it is very easy to overeat another.

6. Eating Too Much Unhealthy Fat

As much as the keto diet is high-fat, consumption of too much of the wrong fats is wrong. Eating too much unsaturated fat should be avoided.

7. Not Drinking Enough Water

It is very easy not to drink enough water, and this is a common mistake by many people, especially newbies to the keto diet. Water is a must for keeping your body healthy while on the journey to ketosis and to maintain it. Dehydration while on ketosis can lead to kidney problems or failure. Put water at the top of your list.

8. Eating Only Animal Products

The efficacy of the keto diet can be misleading if you are not well informed. Include all food types, especially healthy vegetables. Plant foods are important sources of phytonutrients, vitamins, and fiber.

9. Eating Too Much Dairy Products

Consume dairy in moderation of on a keto diet. Dairy products are high in calories, which is counterproductive to what you want. You should burn more calories than you consume.

Forgetting physical exercise

Do not forget as much as the keto diet if efficient at burning fat. Exercise is important while on a ketosis diet to stimulate muscle building and calories and fat burning.

To learn more about this book and how it can help improve your healthy lifestyle, look for the title: "Keto Meal Prep for Beginners: Your Essential Ketogenic Diet Easy Meal Plan to Save Time & Money for Long-Term Weight Loss, Eating Better and Healthy Living" by Amy Maria Adams on the online store.

Conclusion

Thank you again for owning this book!

I hope this book was able to help you to fully grasp what the ketogenic diet is all about. In order to be successful with the diet, the next step is to dutifully execute what you have learned in the book, especially the chapter about the guidelines for getting on the diet.

Thank you and good luck!

www.ingramcontent.com/pod-product-compliance
Lightning Source LLC
Chambersburg PA
CBHW052206090526
44583CB00017BA/2142